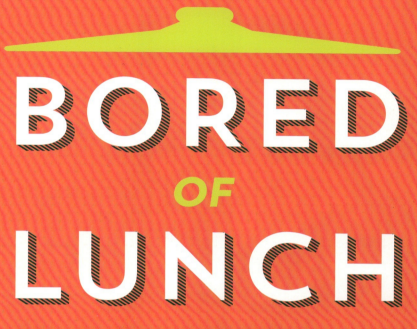

BORED
OF
LUNCH

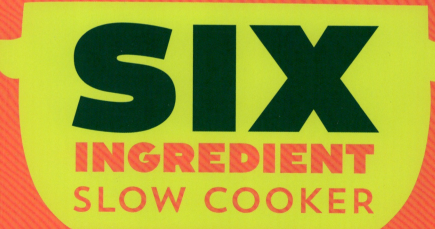

SIX
INGREDIENT
SLOW COOKER

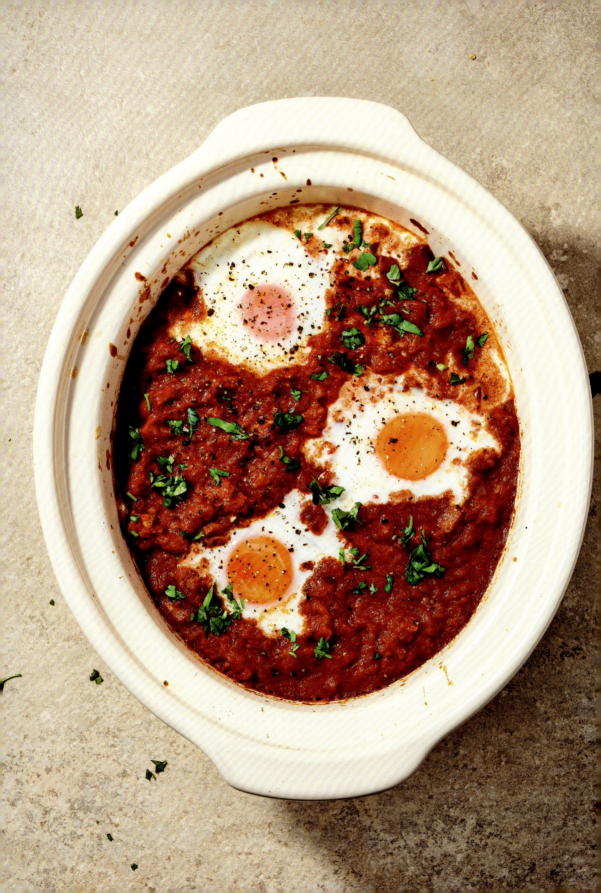

NATHAN ANTHONY

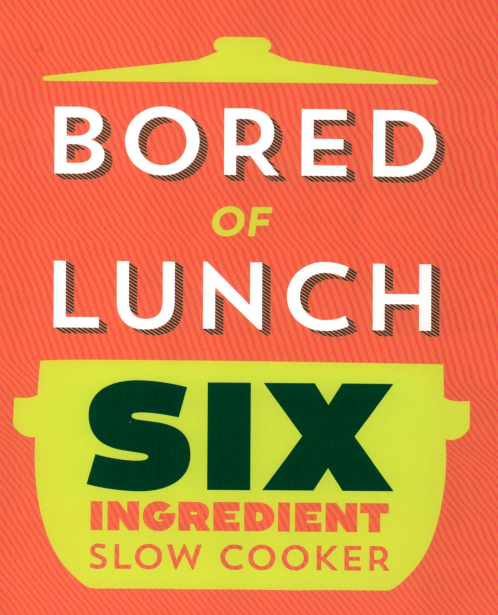

BORED OF LUNCH

OF

SIX INGREDIENT SLOW COOKER

PHOTOGRAPHY BY DAN JONES

EBURY PRESS

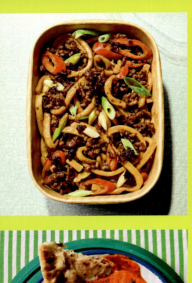
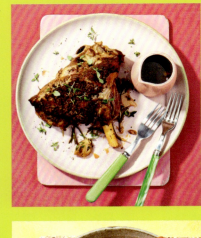
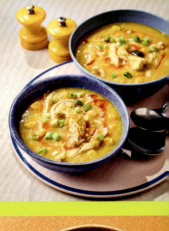
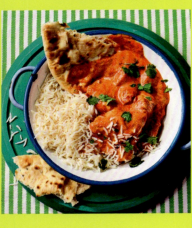
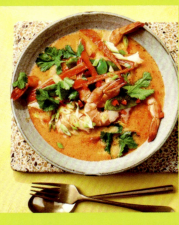
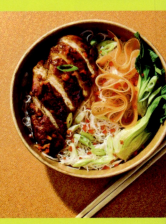
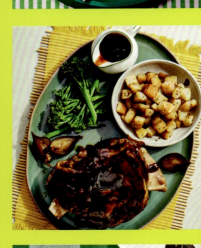
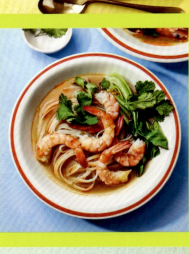
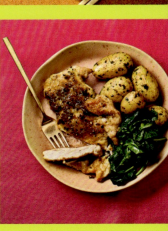
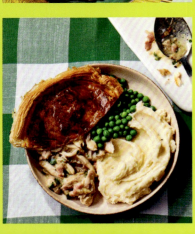
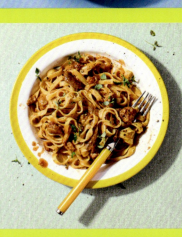
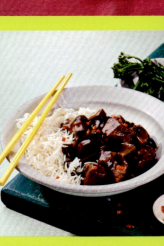

CONTENTS

6   Introduction

8   Pantry essentials

9   Your slow cooker kit

10   6 share & save ingredients

12   How to use this book

14   **FUSS-FREE FAKEAWAYS**

54   **COMFORT FOOD**

84   **SOUPS, LUNCHES & LIGHTER MEALS**

114   **THROW & GO SHARING DINNERS**

146   **SET & FORGET MIDWEEK MEALS**

174   **SIMPLE SWEETS**

186   Index

190   Thanks

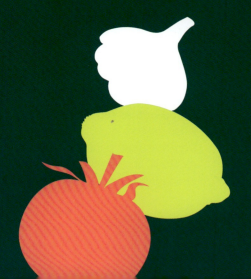

INTRODUCTION

Hello, and welcome to book number five. I actually can't believe we're already at my fifth book, thank you!

Welcome to those of you who are new to Bored of Lunch. I'm Nathan, I'm from Belfast in Northern Ireland, and I'm a busy home cook like you. I have published four international bestselling books so far – two of those are slow cooker books and two are air fryer books. But with this new slow cooker book I want to push boundaries and go with JUST six ingredients for each recipe.

Now, it shouldn't be a shock that I love a kitchen appliance, especially if it's going to save you time, money and effort. I am all about fuss-free, minimal-prep recipes that are full of flavour, so **SIX INGREDIENTS** seemed like the perfect next book for me. There's nothing better than a slow cooker, just stick all your ingredients in – or throw and go, as I like to call it – and let the machine do all the work. Plus, they use less energy than a hob or oven, saving you money in the long run. I've also tried to use super-accessible ingredients in all the recipes, but if there are any you really struggle to find, feel free to swap in other ingredients that you can get more easily.

As this book focuses on using only six ingredients per recipe, you'll see that I have listed the core ingredients but have excluded from these salt, pepper, oil (or butter), water (or stock) and cornflour, as I'm assuming you already have these in your store cupboard (see page 8 for more info on pantry essentials). A note: I've suggested using water in most places because that works perfectly, but I would definitely encourage you to use stock if you have it because it adds so much more flavour. I've also not included the sides or what you serve it with in the six ingredients, partly because you can't cook things like rice or mashed potatoes well in the slow cooker, but mainly because what you serve with your meal is totally up to you. I've added my suggestions, but if you really want to add mash or pasta to your meal, then be my guest.

As with all my previous books, every recipe is calorie-counted, based on the main six ingredients used only. Calories are something I find useful to track, and I know a lot of you have found this helpful in the past, but these books are for you to tailor your recipes to your own specific needs. If you fancy a double portion, or you want to add more ingredients – go ahead! I want you to see these recipes as a base that you can tweak and add to as you see fit. Whether that's adding more veg or cheese or swapping out meat, it's up to you. I know lots of you also love seeing the nutritional breakdown of recipes, so you know you're getting your protein needs and the like – so I've included breakdowns for protein, carbohydrates and fat on all the recipes.

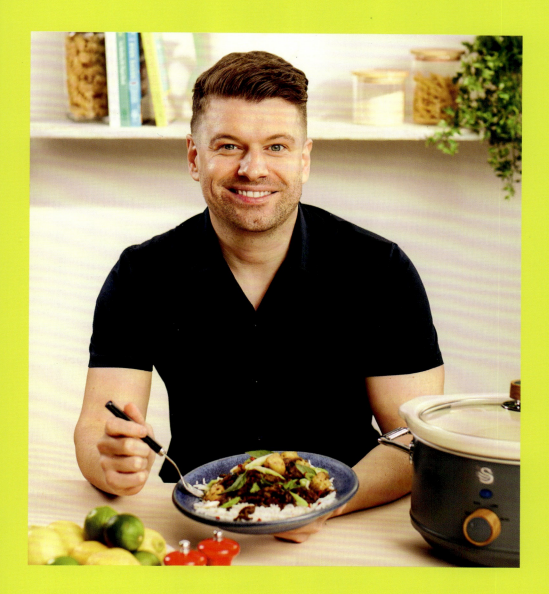

The chapters in this book include the must-have **FUSS-FREE FAKEAWAYS** and **COMFORT FOOD** as well as batch-cook saviours **THROW & GO SHARING DINNERS** and **SET & FORGET MIDWEEK MEALS,** plus easy **SOUPS, LUNCHES & LIGHTER MEALS** and **SIMPLE SWEETS**. I hope you love cooking from this book as much as I've enjoyed writing the recipes. It is stripped-back simplicity at its core and is my favourite book to date. I can't wait to see how you get on with these recipes, so please do share them with me on @boredoflunch. I love seeing you guys making my meals!

Thanks for all your incredible support. Love,

Nathan

PANTRY ESSENTIALS

This book is, of course, very different to my last two slow cooker books, as we use fewer ingredients in each recipe, but there are still lots of ingredients I suggest keeping to hand in your cupboards.

The must-haves are cornflour, for thickening sauces, some oil or butter – although you don't need these for every recipe, and rarely both in the same recipe – then some salt and black pepper and water or stock. As slow cookers need lots of liquid, you should add water or stock to most recipes. In order to not reduce the amount of flavour in the recipes that you can get from other ingredients, I haven't counted water or stock as one of the six ingredients, unless it is essential that you use a certain type of stock in the recipe, such as a rich beef stock. I'd highly encourage you to use stock in your recipes to really maximise the flavour of your meals, but you can just use water if you don't have it to hand or want to save some pennies.

RECIPE MUST-HAVES
- Salt and black pepper
- Cornflour
- Oil or butter
- Water or stock

TINS, JARS & BOTTLES
- Chickpeas
- Beans (borlotti, pinto or cannellini, butter, baked)
- Sweetcorn
- Passata or chopped tomatoes
- Coconut milk
- Dijon mustard
- Pesto
- Honey
- Soy sauce (light and dark)
- Hoisin sauce
- Gochujang paste
- Harissa paste
- Sriracha
- Sweet chilli sauce
- Oyster sauce
- Worcestershire sauce
- White wine (and white wine vinegar)
- Red wine

FRESH
- Coriander leaves
- Parsley
- Garlic
- Ginger (plus garlic and ginger paste)
- Basil
- Thyme
- Sage
- Oregano
- Curry leaves
- Potatoes
- Onions
- Lemons, limes and oranges
- Chillies (red and green)
- Spring onions

LONG LIFE
- Curry pastes and powders of your choice
- Seasoning packets (e.g. Cajun, taco)
- Sesame seeds
- Ground cumin, coriander and cinnamon, dried thyme, basil and oregano – and dried mixed herbs
- Paprika
- Chilli flakes
- Cinnamon sticks
- Rice (e.g. basmati, jasmine)
- Couscous
- Dried pasta (e.g. penne, fusilli)
- Tomato purée
- Flour (plain and self-raising)
- Stocks, including vegetable, chicken, lamb, fish, beef and rich beef (*stock pots, cubes or fresh*)
- Cocoa powder
- Caster sugar
- Soft light brown sugar

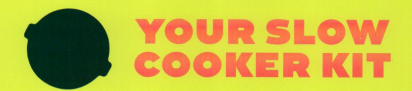

YOUR SLOW COOKER KIT

I use a 3.5-litre slow cooker, which will work for all the recipes. The items listed below are optional, as you can make all of the recipes in this book without having to use any of them, but while the slow cooker will do everything you need, these are helpful to have for various reasons.

I. SILICONE LINERS

These can sometimes help to prevent meat or sauces drying out – such as a turkey crown – but they also prevent the pot getting as messy and make washing up easier.

2. PLASTIC LINERS

I know a lot of my online followers use these, which are perfect for the recipes that are steepers and leave a mess. Simply add a liner to a slow cooker before adding the ingredients, then remove once you've finished and you have a clean pot you don't have to scrub afterwards.

3. ZIPLOC BAGS

These are perfect for prepping ahead; you can throw your six ingredients into a bag and place in the fridge or freezer until ready to use. Then simply empty the contents into your slow cooker, switch it on and go about your day while it bubbles away. I prefer the reusable ones as they are better for the environment – just wash and reuse.

4. MEAT THERMOMETER

Not essential, but if you are cooking large cuts of meat like a whole chicken or a pork roast, these will help you make sure the meat is cooked through and just as you like it.

6 SHARE & SAVE INGREDIENTS

When cooking meals, I often find I open a packet of something for a recipe and then have some left over, usually some chicken or cheese. I never want to let ingredients go to waste, so here I've suggested the six most used ingredients and recipes where they share the same ingredients. This will help you to reduce waste and save you money, too.

CRÈME FRAÎCHE

Simple Steak Diane
(page 68)

Pesto & Sundried Tomato Chicken
(page 71)

Creamy Pork Sausage Pasta
(page 76)

Creamy White Wine Chicken
(page 79)

Lemon Paprika Cod
(page 139)

Creamy Beef & Mushroom Orzotto
(page 140)

Lazy Chicken Stroganoff
(page 168)

DOUBLE CREAM

Creamy Chicken Pasta with Mushrooms & Bacon
(page 63)

Winter Sausage Meatballs & Cream
(page 66)

Garlic Butter Chicken with Bacon & Sweetcorn
(page 80)

Broccoli, Leek & Stilton Soup
(page 96)

Creamy Chicken & Potato Soup
(page 98)

Black Lentil Dahl
(page 101)

Marry Me Chicken Made Easy
(page 148)

Creamy Chicken Meatballs with Gnocchi
(page 150)

Creamy Butternut Squash & Lemon Linguine
(page 160)

CHORIZO

Chorizo & Butter Bean Soup
(page 93)

Harissa & Chorizo Shakshuka
(page 104)

Curried Chorizo, Bacon & Lentil Soup
(page 112)

Chickpea, Potato & Chorizo Stew
(page 156)

CHICKEN
(BREASTS OR THIGHS)

Chicken Biryani
(page 16)

Honey & Sriracha Chicken
(page 24)

Takeaway-inspired Garlic Pepper Chicken
(page 34)

Easy Ramen
(page 40)

Chicken Chasni Curry
(page 42)

Pesto & Sundried Tomato Chicken
(page 71)

Garlic Butter Chicken with Bacon & Sweetcorn
(page 80)

Creamy White Wine Chicken
(page 79)

Creamy Chicken & Potato Soup
(page 98)

Chicken & Sweetcorn Soup
(page 109)

Chicken & Bean White Chilli
(page 123)

Honey BBQ Shredded Chicken Burgers
(page 126)

Marry Me Chicken Made Easy
(page 148)

Tomato, Bacon & Basil Chicken Pasta
(page 155)

Lemon, Black Pepper & Butter Chicken
(page 163)

Lazy Chicken Stroganoff
(page 168)

CHEDDAR CHEESE

Philly Cheesesteak Rolls
(page 23)

Cheesy Jalapeño Mince
(page 72)

Cheesy Beef Taco-style Rice
(page 131)

Meatball Sub Bake with Crispy Croutons
(page 166)

STREAKY BACON

Chicken & Bacon Pie
(page 56)

Creamy Chicken Pasta with Mushrooms & Bacon
(page 63)

Beef & Bacon Hotpot
(page 74)

Garlic Butter Chicken with Bacon & Sweetcorn
(page 80)

Chunky Bacon, Leek & Potato Soup
(page 102)

Curried Chorizo, Bacon & Lentil Soup
(page 112)

Tomato, Bacon & Basil Chicken Pasta
(page 155)

Sausage, Bacon & Bean Cowboy Supper
(page 171)

HOW TO USE THIS BOOK

The recipes in this book have each been designed around six ingredients, to make cooking as fuss-free and easy as possible and, in particular, to reduce the amount of planning required.

To help with this, I've included some handy symbols so you can see at a glance if a recipe is suitable for freezing, if it's veggie, and the hands-on prep time (depending on how fast you chop!).

 PREP TIME

 FREEZABLE

 VEGETARIAN

When it comes to freezing and defrosting cooked food, the important thing is to ensure it has cooled to room temperature before putting it in the freezer, and to make sure you reheat everything thoroughly until it's piping hot throughout. Do not refreeze food that has already been defrosted once. However, if you've defrosted raw meat/fish, you can cook it and then freeze it.

I've included a list of my pantry essentials – the ingredients I find most helpful to have in my cupboard – on page 8.

A healthy balance and a note on calories – I don't come from a fitness background and I'm not a nutritionist, but I do track my calories to suit my nutritional needs and goals. There are lots of apps that will recommend your ideal calorie intake based on your height and weight (as a general guide, the NHS recommends 2,000 calories per day for women and 2,500 for men). Each recipe has a nutritional breakdown to show calories, protein, carbohydrates and fat per serving, so this book can be useful for you if you're trying to tailor your diet to a specific target, while still leaving you plenty of room for snacks throughout the day. However, if calorie counting isn't something that's important to you, feel free to make swaps that suit you.

Finally, if a side or serving suggestion has been included in the serving note or method (such as rice, pasta, noodles and veg), this will not be included in the final calorie count. If I've listed something as optional (including optional serving suggestions), this isn't included in the total either. This is so you can see the calorie content of the core six ingredients, then add your sides as you like.

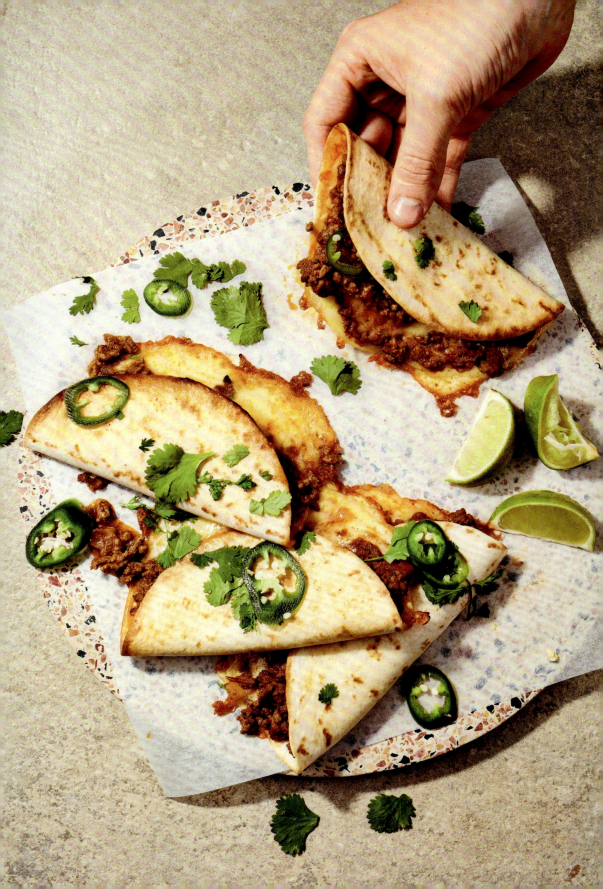

FUSS-FREE
FAKE-AWAYS

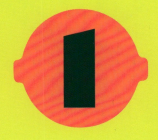

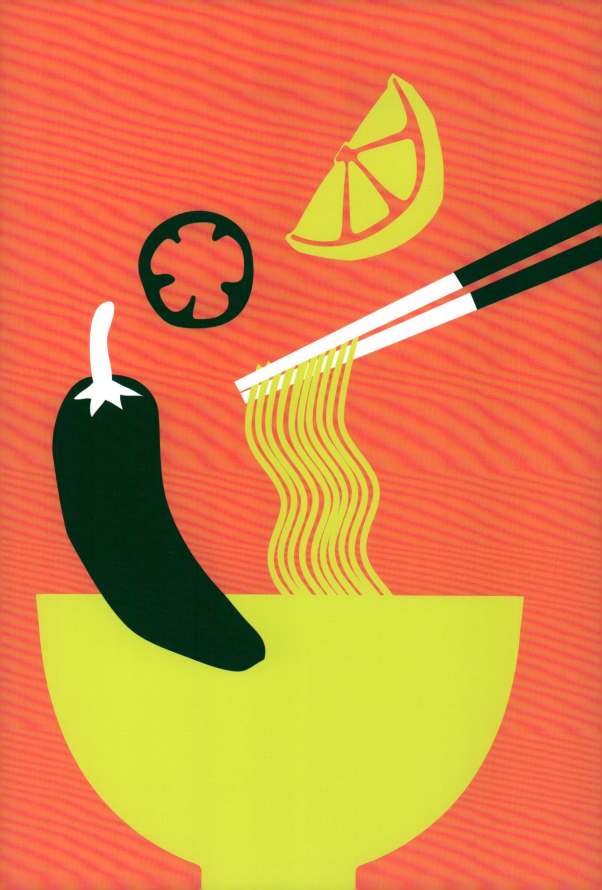

CHICKEN BIRYANI

500 CALORIES

SERVES 4

5 MINS

We're starting the book with a simple one-pot classic that involves throwing everything in, even the rice. You can play around with your favourite curry paste here, but whatever you choose, you won't be disappointed.

500g chicken breasts, diced

6 tbsp curry paste (I love balti with this one)

1 onion, finely diced

handful of fresh coriander, roughly chopped, plus extra to garnish

250g white basmati rice

80g golden raisins

1 Coat the chicken pieces in 2 tablespoons of the curry paste, then cook in a frying pan in 1 tablespoon of oil for 1–2 minutes over a medium heat. Add to the slow cooker with the onion, remaining curry paste, the chopped coriander and 100ml of boiling water or stock and season well with salt and pepper.

2 Cook on high for 2 hours or low for 4 hours. Add in the rice, raisins and 650ml of boiling water or stock. Cook on high for a further 1 hour, then scatter over some extra coriander to garnish, and serve.

PROTEIN: 37g | **CARBS:** 72g | **FAT:** 9g

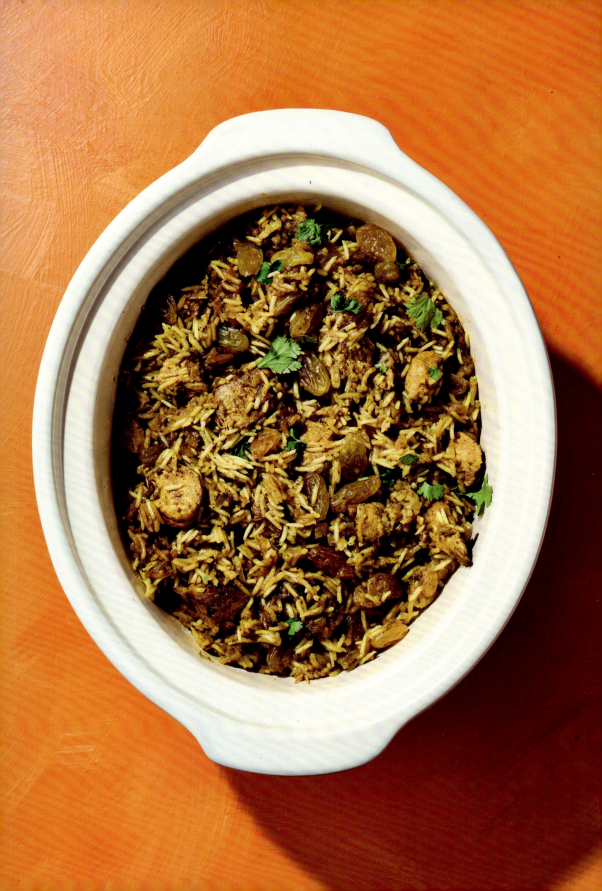

TANGY LEMONGRASS PORK

243 CALORIES

SERVES 4

10 MINS

The first time I tried this dish was while staying in London about to do my first ever LIVE TV appearance on *This Morning*. I was slightly nervous and wanted to revise and prep in my room, so I got a Vietnamese takeaway.

600g boneless pork shoulder, sliced into thin-ish strips

2–3 tbsp chopped lemongrass (or lemongrass purée or paste)

3 garlic cloves, crushed

1 tbsp soft light brown sugar or honey

5 tbsp dark soy sauce

1 tbsp fish sauce

1   Briefly fry the pork in 1 tablespoon of a nut-based oil in a frying pan over a medium heat until browned all over.

2   Add the browned pork to the slow cooker with all the other ingredients and cook on high for 3–4 hours or low for 6–7 hours.

3   Serve with sides of your choice.

SERVING NOTE:
I love serving this with rice noodles and a salad with some lime wedges for squeezing over and topped with finely diced red chilli.

TIP: *You can use any cut of meat here, including beef or chicken thigh fillets.*

PROTEIN: 33g | **CARBS:** 7g | **FAT:** 9g

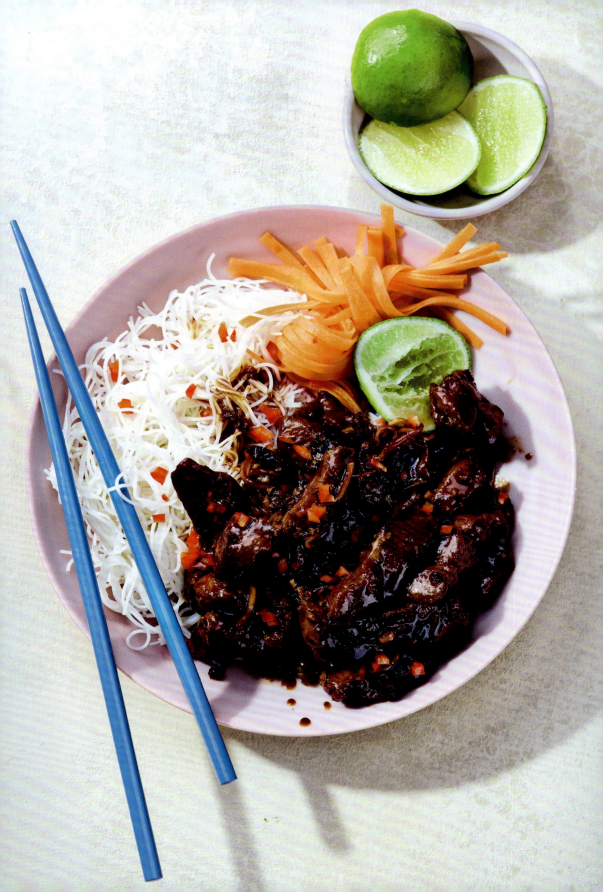

BEEF BRISKET COCONUT RENDANG CURRY

483 CALORIES

SERVES 4

10 MINS

I love a curry and this one will blow you away. It's super-simple and packed with a nutty, buttery sweetness from the coconut milk. What more could you want?

600g beef brisket, unrolled

150g rendang paste

400ml tin of reduced-fat coconut milk

50g desiccated coconut

4 dried makrut lime leaves or curry leaves

5 green cardamom pods, whole

1 Season the brisket with salt and pepper, then add a tablespoon of oil to a large frying pan and sear the meat over a medium heat on all sides until sealed.

2 Transfer to the slow cooker with all the other ingredients and 100ml of boiling water or beef stock. Cook on high for 4 hours or low for 8 hours until the beef is cooked and completely tender.

3 Shred the meat using two forks in the pot, or, if you prefer, carefully remove the brisket from the sauce to a plate to do this, then return the beef to the pot and stir to coat the meat. Remove the cardamom pods (and curry leaves, if you want) from the curry sauce.

4 Serve hot with your preferred side dish.

SERVING NOTE:
This pairs perfectly with some rice and fresh coriander sprinkled over.

PROTEIN: 35g | **CARBS:** 7g | **FAT:** 35g

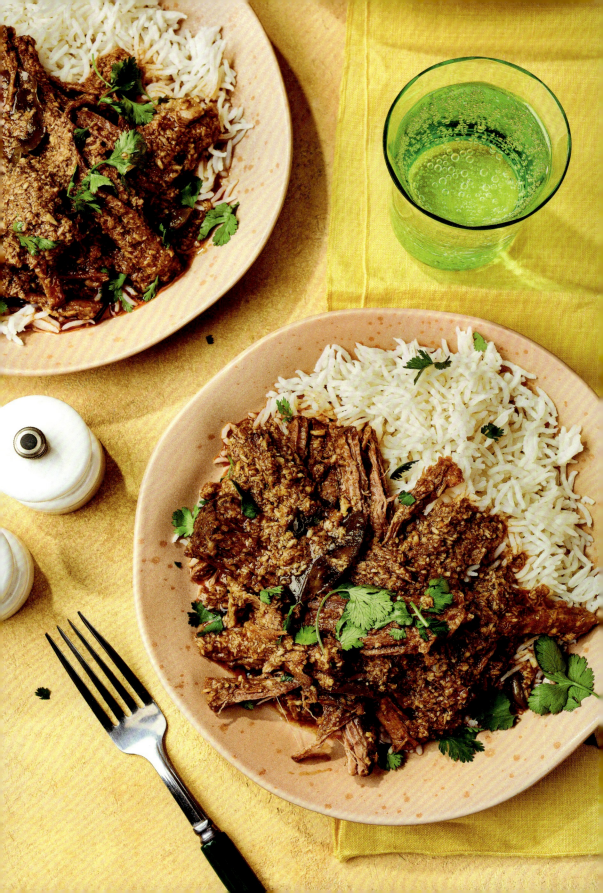

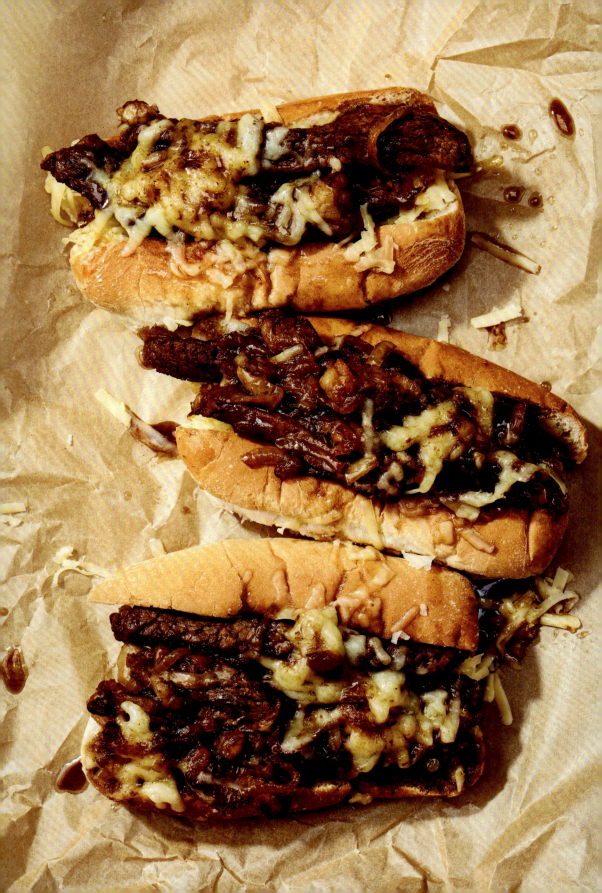

PHILLY CHEESESTEAK ROLLS

545 CALORIES

SERVES 4

15 MINS

Call this the tidier version of a Sloppy Joe – messy, but not as sloppy. It's a beef steak that's lightly seasoned and cooked until falling apart, then paired with cheese and onions in a bread roll. Heaven! I love adding mustard, but it's not essential.

600g beef steak (rump or sirloin)

3 onions, sliced

2 tbsp white wine vinegar

3 tbsp Worcestershire sauce

4 bread rolls

150g reduced-fat Cheddar cheese, grated

1 Season the steak with salt and pepper. Pan-fry the steak over a medium heat in 2 tablespoons of oil for 2 minutes on each side, then remove from the pan and set aside. Soften the onions in the remaining oil.

2 Cut the steak into strips and add to the slow cooker with the softened onions and pan juices, as well as the vinegar and Worcestershire sauce. Cook on high for 3 hours or low for 6 hours.

3 Slice in half and then toast your bread rolls, fill them with the beef mixture, sprinkle over the cheese and top with your sauce of choice, if you like – but these are so good you won't need any.

TIP: *For extra saucy rolls, add some ketchup and a dash of mustard.*

PROTEIN: 52g | **CARBS:** 43g | **FAT:** 19g

HONEY & SRIRACHA CHICKEN

280 CALORIES

SERVES 4

5 MINS

This recipe is a prime example of why the Fakeaways chapter is my favourite – lazy, but loaded with flavour. It's an incredible dish for cutting corners and saves so much prep time, but it still wows on taste. I prefer to seal the chicken before slow-cooking it, for extra flavour, but you can skip this step if you prefer.

4 chicken breasts, whole

6 tbsp sriracha

4 tbsp honey

juice of 1 lemon

3 garlic cloves, grated

1 tbsp dark soy sauce

1 Coat the chicken breasts all over in 1 tablespoon of cornflour, then pan-fry over a medium heat in 1 tablespoon of hot oil for 2 minutes, or until golden on both sides.

2 Transfer the chicken to the slow cooker with all the other ingredients. Cook on high for 3 hours or low for 6 hours.

3 Slice and serve the chicken breasts.

SERVING NOTE:
This is great served with rice noodles, pak choi, carrots, some spring onions and chopped red chilli.

TIP: *You can skip pan-frying the chicken beforehand; the texture will just be a bit different.*

PROTEIN: 36g | **CARBS:** 23g | **FAT:** 5g

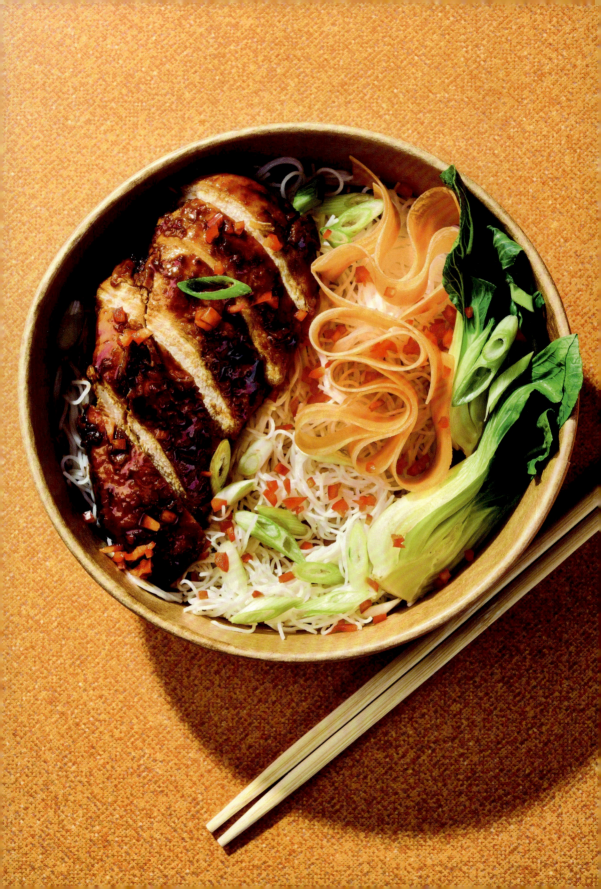

EASY BEEF & MUSHROOMS IN OYSTER SAUCE

243 CALORIES

SERVES 4

5 MINS

If you automatically think fish when you see the word oyster, fear not – this will not taste like a fish dish; it's tender beef and mushrooms in a gorgeous, sweet and flavoursome sauce that anyone can make. It's beyond simple.

600g beef steaks, cut into chunks

200g chestnut mushrooms, quartered or halved

4 tbsp oyster sauce

3 tbsp sweet chilli sauce

4 tbsp dark soy sauce

1 tbsp ginger purée

1 Add all the ingredients to the slow cooker along with some pepper and 1 tablespoon of cornflour mixed with 1 tablespoon of water. Cook on high for 3–4 hours or low for 5–6 hours.

2 Serve!

SERVING NOTE:
Rice and green veg (Tenderstem broccoli or pak choi) work well. I like to scatter over a little chopped red chilli too.

PROTEIN: 35g | **CARBS:** 12g | **FAT:** 7g

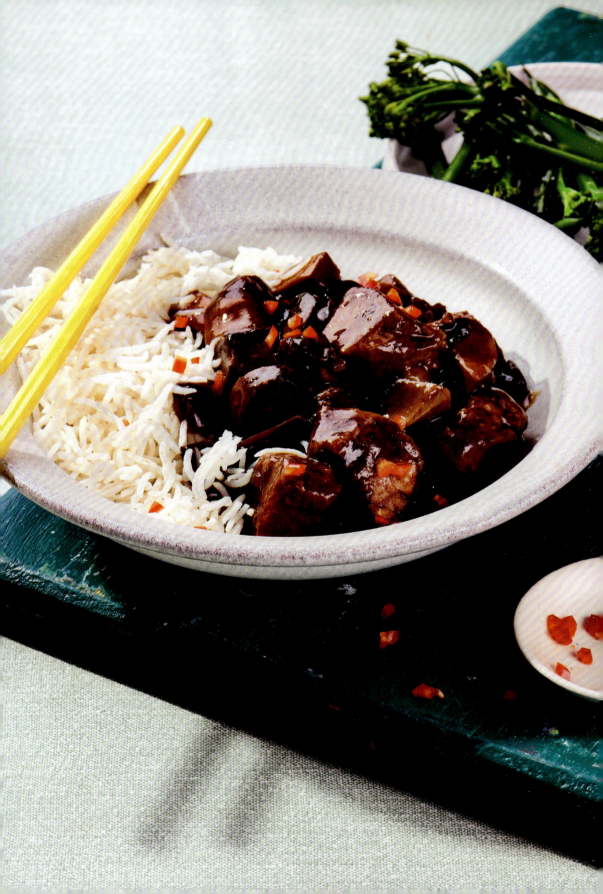

KING PRAWN CURRY

183 CALORIES

SERVES 4

5 MINS

This effortlessly creamy prawn curry will create a party in your mouth. The key to maximum flavour with minimal ingredients is simply using your favourite curry paste.

400g large raw prawns, peeled

4 tbsp balti curry paste

400ml tin of reduced-fat coconut milk

1 tbsp garlic and ginger paste

grated zest and juice of 2 limes, plus lime wedges for squeezing over

2 cinnamon sticks

1 Add everything to the slow cooker and cook on high for 3 hours or low for 6 hours.

2 Remove the cinnamon sticks (if you want). If the sauce looks a bit thin, thicken it with 3 tablespoons of water mixed with 1 tablespoon of cornflour, then season with salt and pepper.

3 Serve.

SERVING NOTE:
Goes well with noodles or rice and a squeeze of lime.

TIP: *You can use any curry paste of your choice here.*

PROTEIN: 10g | **CARBS:** 4g | **FAT:** 10g

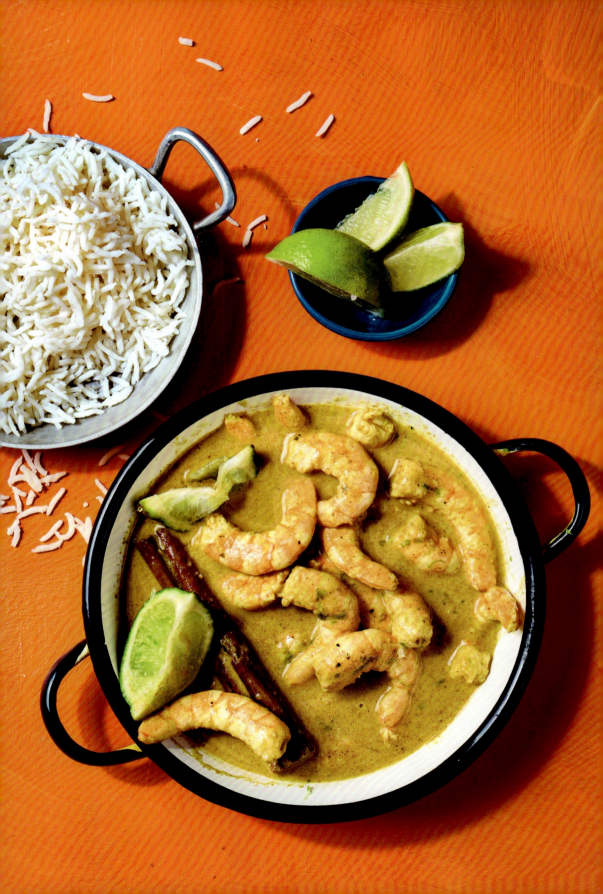

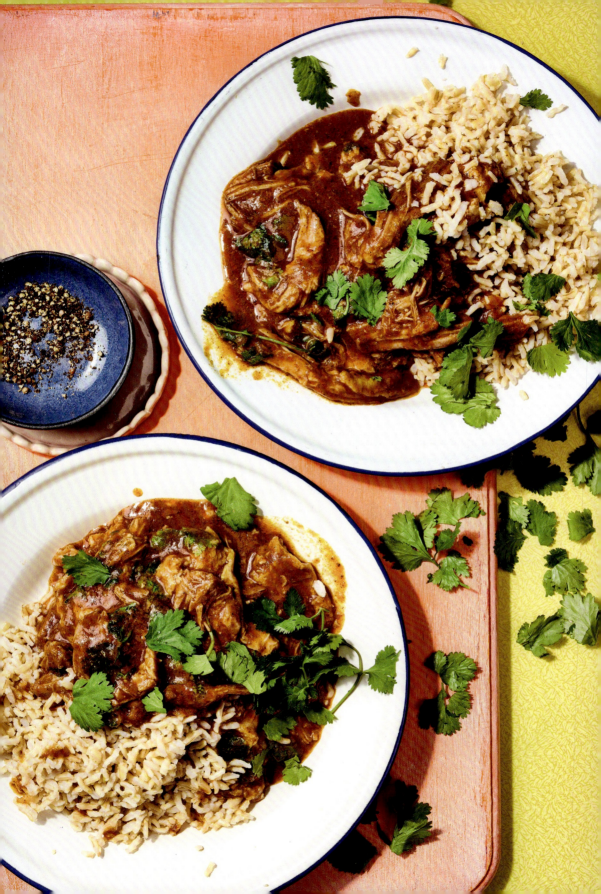

ROGAN JOSH PULLED PORK CURRY

345 CALORIES

SERVES 6

5 MINS

A super simple dish that packs one hell of a punch, finished with coconut milk stirred through to give you all the creamy rogan josh feels, but without all those extra calories. I could eat this over and over again and never tire of it.

1.2kg boneless pork shoulder

4 tbsp rogan josh curry paste

400g passata

handful of fresh coriander, roughly chopped, plus extra to serve

1 cinnamon stick

400ml tin of reduced-fat coconut milk

1 Massage the pork joint all over in 1–2 tablespoons of the curry paste.

2 Add the remaining paste to the slow cooker with 50ml of boiling water and all the other ingredients, except the coconut milk. Cook on high for 6–8 hours or low for 10–12 hours.

3 Before the last 30 minutes of cooking, season with salt and pepper, stir through the coconut milk, discard the cinnamon stick and shred the pork in the pot using two forks.

4 Serve with extra coriander sprinkled over.

SERVING NOTE:
Rice works well with this.

PROTEIN: 45g | **CARBS:** 6g | **FAT:** 15g

GOCHUJANG & BBQ PULLED BEEF

281 CALORIES

SERVES 6

5 MINS

I don't think you can make a fakeaway with as little fuss as this. Almost no chopping needed, throw it all in and carry on with the rest of your day. Then, return to a gorgeous Korean-inspired pulled beef that's perfect served with tacos and slaw or rice – my preference is some rice with some finely chopped red chilli for a bit more heat.

1kg beef brisket, unrolled

400g passata

4 tbsp BBQ sauce

2 tbsp gochujang paste

2 red chillies, finely diced, plus extra to serve

2 tbsp dark soy sauce

1   Add all the ingredients to the slow cooker with some salt and pepper and 200ml of boiling water, then cook on high for 4–5 hours or low for 8–9 hours.

2   Shred the beef in the pot using two forks and scatter over the remaining chopped red chilli.

PROTEIN: 36g | **CARBS:** 11g | **FAT:** 10g

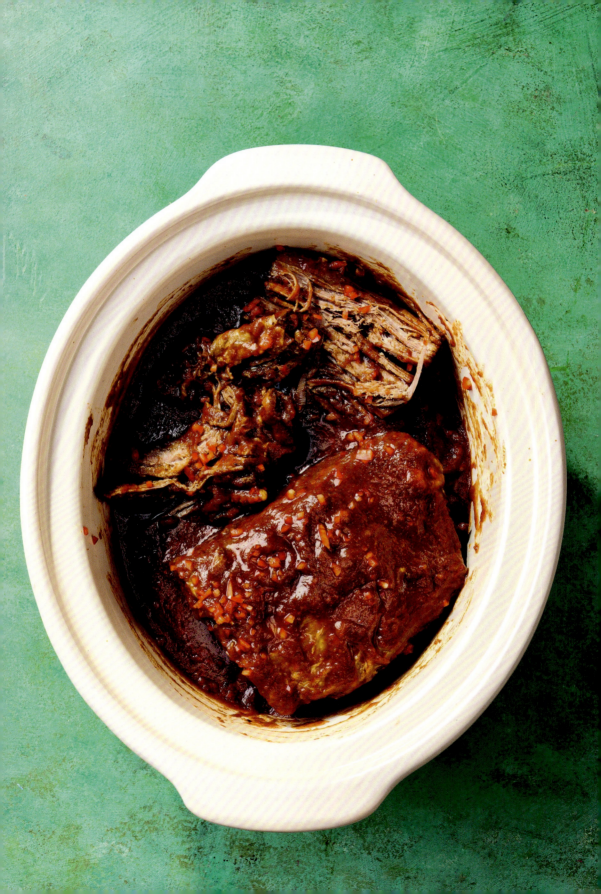

TAKEAWAY-INSPIRED GARLIC PEPPER CHICKEN

246 CALORIES

SERVES 4

5 MINS

I'm honestly not sure how something so easy can taste so incredibly good. This is inspired by my travels to Thailand, and I must warn you, if garlic isn't your thing, this might not be for you. Traditionally, this uses a whole bulb of confit garlic, and I am all for it.

500g boneless and skinless chicken thighs, whole

3 tbsp garlic purée

5 tbsp light soy sauce

3 tbsp oyster sauce

juice of 1 lime, plus 1 lime cut into wedges to serve

3 tbsp honey

1 There isn't really a method with this, just throw it all in and cook on high for 3 hours or low for 6 hours. Partway through cooking, check and add good amount of pepper and a splash of water to the mix if it looks a little dry.

2 Serve with any sides you fancy and lime wedges for squeezing over.

SERVING NOTE:
This goes great with noodles, fresh coriander leaves and some lime wedges. I love to use the remaining sauce as a dipping sauce, too!

PROTEIN: 28g | **CARBS:** 19g | **FAT:** 7g

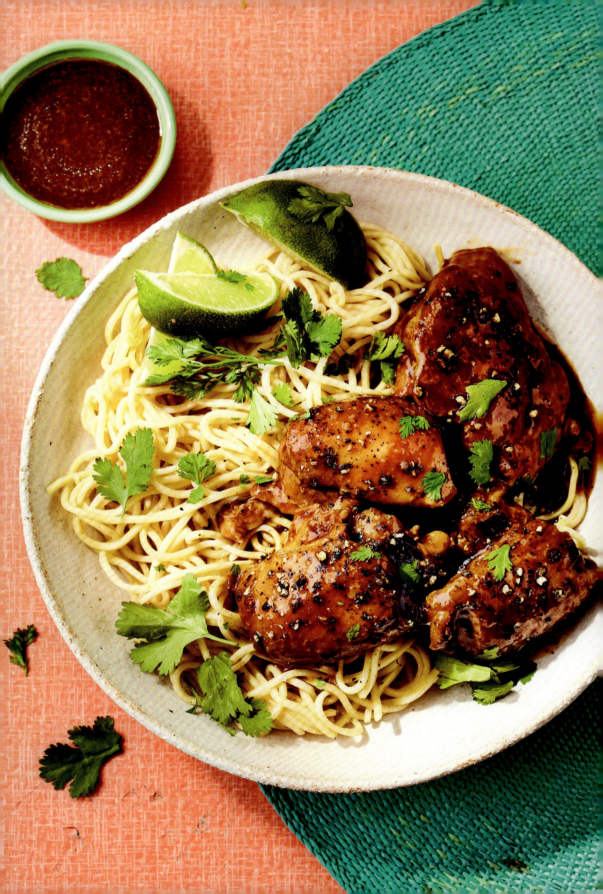

SAUSAGE CURRYWURST

268 CALORIES

SERVES 4

5 MINS

Divine, iconic, German street food in a slow cooker – your palate is going to go on all sorts of adventures here. You can load this with as many flavours as you like, but simplicity always wins – and so does this six-ingredient version.

8 frankfurter sausages (or your favourite pork sausages)

2–3 tbsp mild curry powder

2 tbsp yellow mustard

1 tbsp Worcestershire sauce

400g passata

1 tbsp apple cider vinegar

1 Add all the ingredients, some salt and pepper and 50ml of boiling water to the slow cooker. Cook on high for 4 hours or low for 7–8 hours.

2 Once cooked, remove the sausages and cut them into small slices/chunks and then finish with that beaut sauce.

SERVING NOTE:
A great excuse to use your air fryer – make some air-fried chips and serve with the sausages.

PROTEIN: 11g | **CARBS:** 12g | **FAT:** 19g

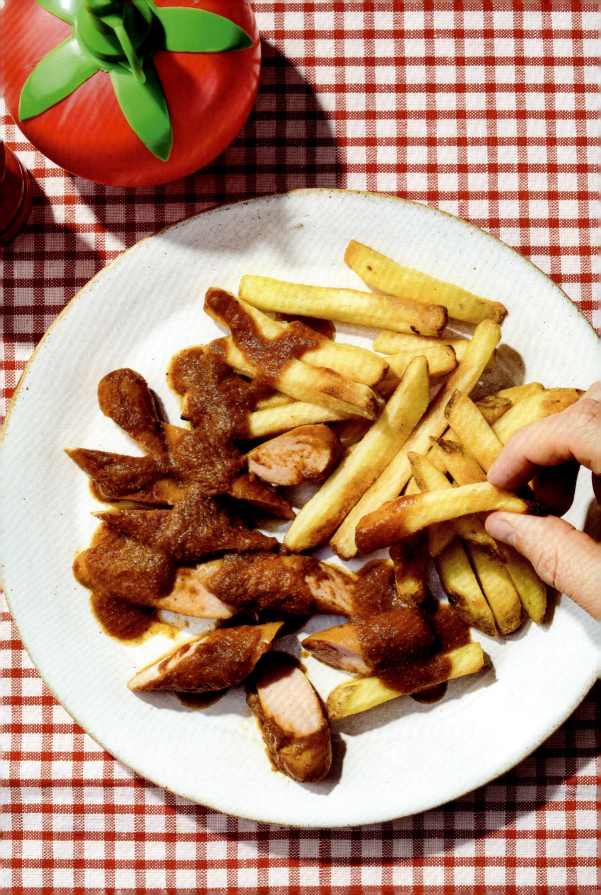

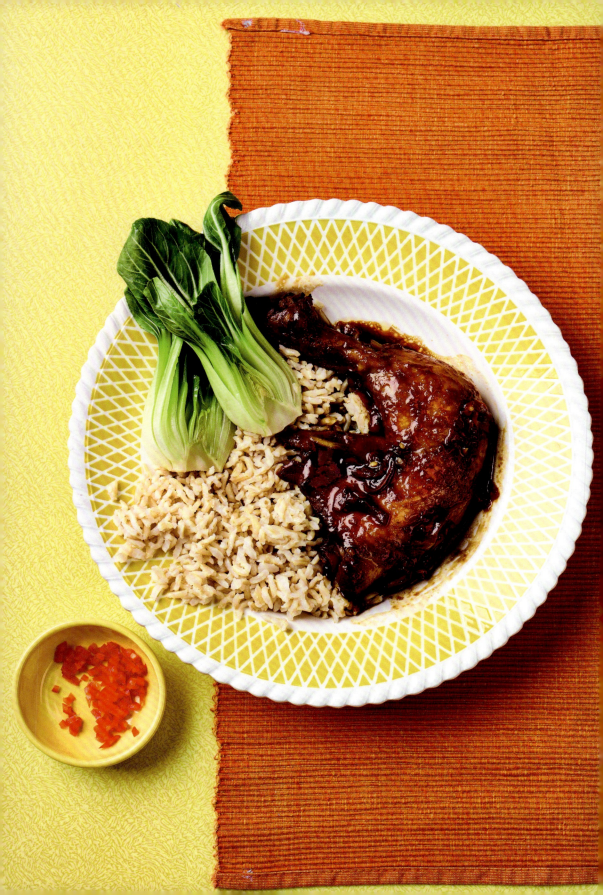

STICKY HOISIN & ORANGE CHICKEN LEGS

156 CALORIES

SERVES 4

5 MINS

The recipe title does all the talking here, so I don't even need to explain it. Chicken meat that falls off the bone in a zingy sticky sauce, paired perfectly with rice and pak choi.

4 chicken legs, skin on

4 tbsp hoisin sauce

3 tbsp light soy sauce

1 red chilli, finely diced, plus extra finely chopped, to serve

juice of 1 large orange

3 garlic cloves, crushed

1 Add all the ingredients to the slow cooker with some pepper. Cook on high for 4 hours or low for 8 hours.

2 Serve with sides of your choice!

SERVING NOTE:
Serve the chicken legs with rice, pak choi and a little extra chopped chilli.

PROTEIN: 17g | **CARBS:** 12g | **FAT:** 5g

EASY RAMEN

815 CALORIES

SERVES 2

5 MINS

Ramen, the easy way! The basic recipe uses just six ingredients, but if you like you can change it up by serving with any of the optional extras listed below.

1 litre ramen broth (I like tonkotsu or chicken)

2 tbsp white miso paste

400g boneless and skinless chicken thighs or pork belly, sliced

300g dried ramen noodles

1 tbsp light soy sauce, plus extra to taste (optional)

225g tin of bamboo shoots, drained

1 Pour a little broth into a small bowl and whisk in the miso paste, then add this to the slow cooker along with the rest of the broth. Add the meat and cook on high for 2 hours or low for 4 hours. Once the meat is completely tender, you can leave it in the broth or remove it and grill it under a high heat briefly to crisp it up.

2 Add the noodles, soy sauce and bamboo shoots to the broth in the slow cooker, pop the lid on and cook on high for 30 minutes, or until the noodles are cooked through.

3 Taste for seasoning and add more soy sauce if needed. Return the meat to the dish if you have grilled it, then serve in large bowls.

SERVING NOTE:

You could bulk out this meal and serve with halved boiled eggs, scattered with black sesame seeds, sliced spring onions and some chilli oil.

PROTEIN: 71g | **CARBS:** 104g | **FAT:** 12g

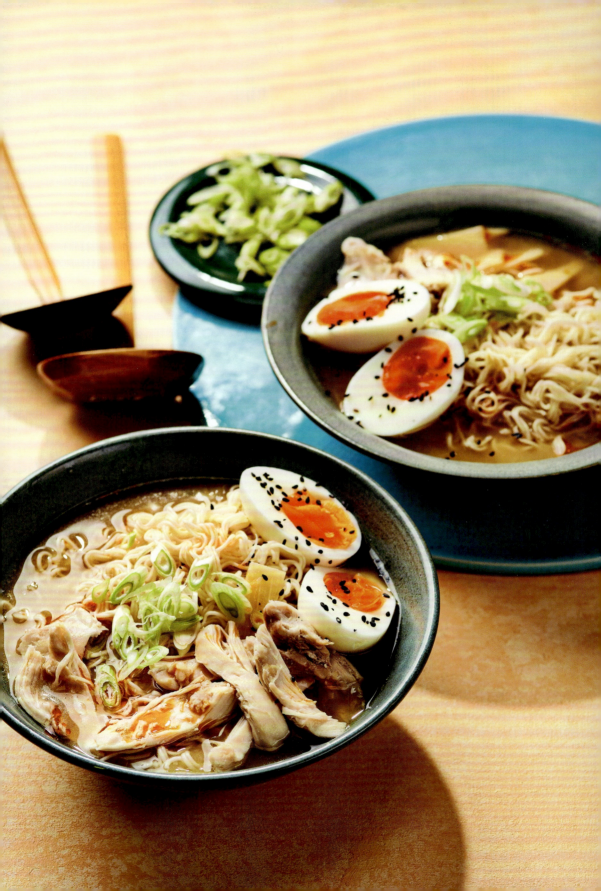

CHICKEN CHASNI CURRY

176 CALORIES

SERVES 4

5 MINS

You can add every spice you have to this gorgeous curry, if you like, but the simplicity of this stripped-back six-ingredient version hits the spot and is incredibly budget-friendly. You can use chicken thighs here, if you prefer, and add some veg, too.

400g chicken breasts, diced

3 tbsp chicken tikka paste

500g passata

2 tsp red food colouring

1 tbsp garlic and ginger paste

1 tbsp mango chutney

1 Add all the ingredients to the slow cooker with some salt and pepper. Cook on high for 3 hours or low for 6 hours.

2 If you fancy, stir in 2–3 tablespoons of double cream just before serving and top with chopped coriander.

SERVING NOTE:
This goes really well with some naan bread for dipping into the sauce.

PROTEIN: 23g | **CARBS:** 10g | **FAT:** 4g

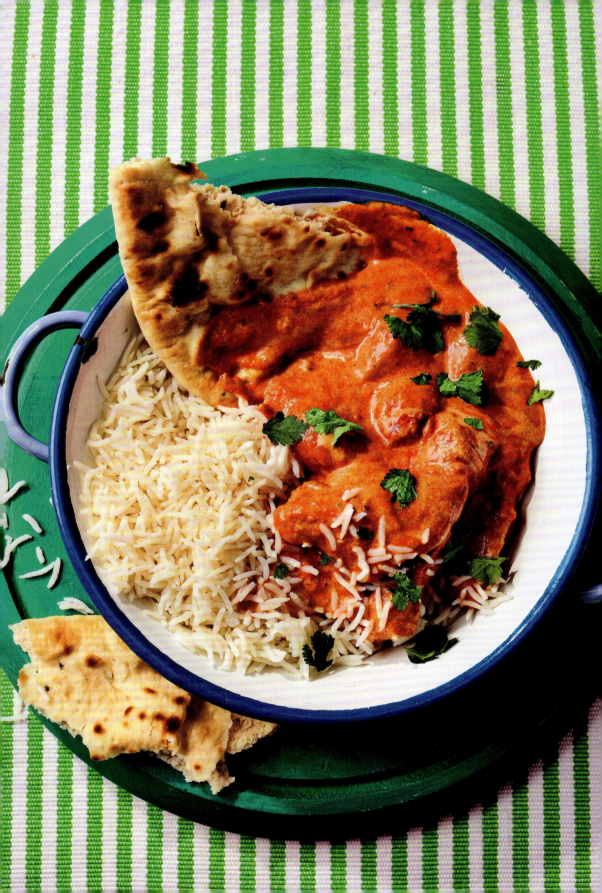

STICKY CHILLI MINCE & NOODLES

465 CALORIES

SERVES 4

10 MINS

Once you start making this Dan Dan Noodles inspired dish, you won't stop. It's a sticky, sweet chilli mince served with your favourite noodles. Honey, a good dash of mild chilli flakes and a nutty flavour from the peanut butter combine to make a true power trio.

500g lean beef or pork mince

4 tbsp light soy sauce

1 tsp chilli flakes

4 tbsp honey

2 tbsp smooth peanut butter or tahini

125g cooked noodles per person (I like udon)

1 Fry the mince in a pan with 1 tablespoon of your preferred oil (I like sesame oil here) for 2–3 minutes over a medium heat until browned.

2 Add the browned mince to the slow cooker with all the other ingredients, except the cooked noodles. Season with some black pepper, then cook on high for 3–4 hours or low for 6–7 hours.

3 Stir in the cooked noodles and ENJOY – it is delicious. If you prefer more sauce, you can add a tablespoon of water.

SERVING NOTE:
For even more flavour, add a squeeze of lime juice when you serve this and scatter with some sliced spring onion and red chilli.

TIP: *You could swap in Chinese 5 spice for the chilli flakes.*

PROTEIN: 34g | **CARBS:** 48g | **FAT:** 14g

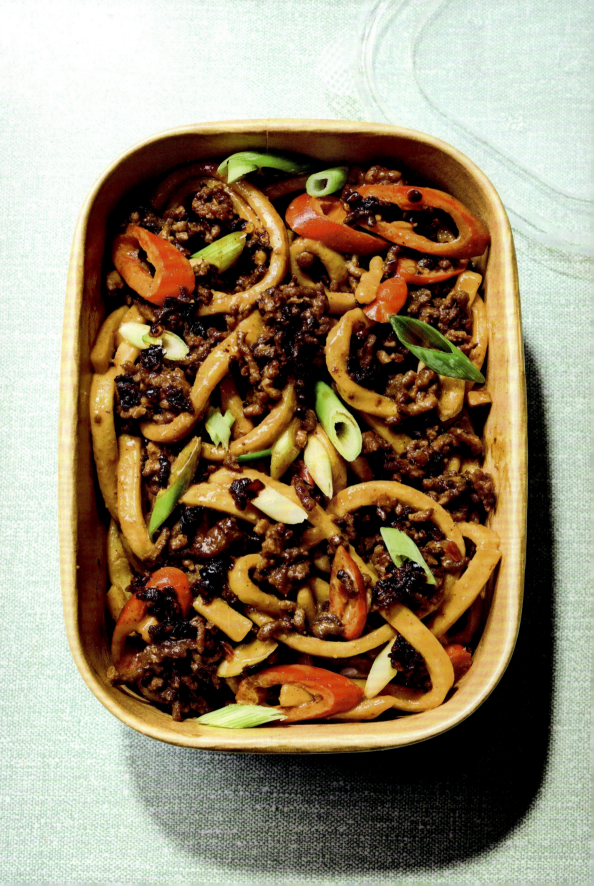

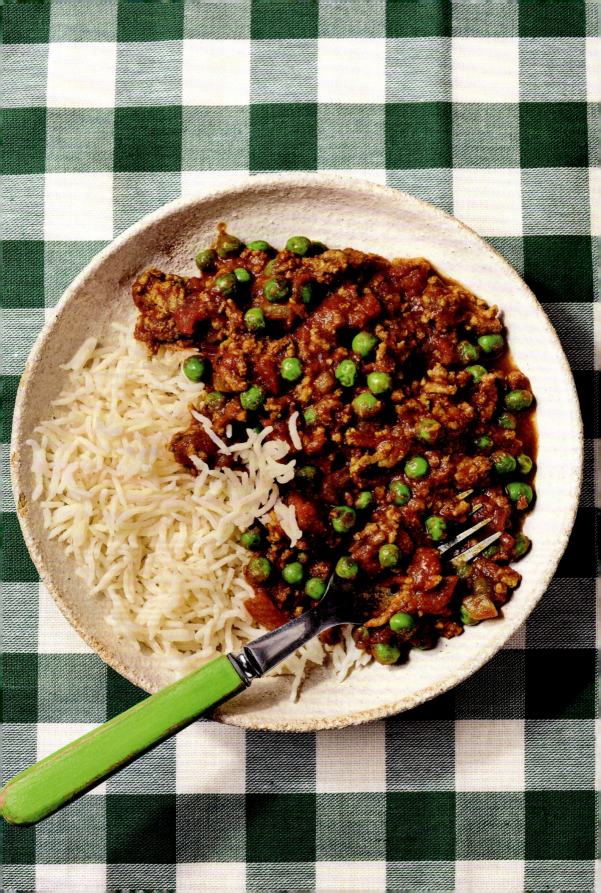

LAMB KEEMA

SERVES 4

10 MINS

One ingredient I get asked for help to be creative with is mince. This impressive fakeaway does just that, combining flavourful lamb mince with frozen peas and the spices of a mild curry. It is divine.

400g lean lamb mince

1 onion, finely chopped

2 x 400g tins of chopped tomatoes

4 tbsp rogan josh curry paste

1 tbsp garlic and ginger paste

200g frozen peas

1 If you have time, brown the mince in a frying pan with 1 tablespoon of oil over a medium heat, then add it to the slow cooker with all the other ingredients, except the peas. Add some salt and pepper and 150ml of boiling water. Cook on high for 3–4 hours or low for 7–8 hours.

2 Stir in the frozen peas and cook for the last 30 minutes.

3 Serve.

SERVING NOTE:
This goes great with freshly cooked fluffy rice.

PROTEIN: 25g | **CARBS:** 17g | **FAT:** 18g

DUCK LEGS & PINEAPPLE CURRY

676 CALORIES

SERVES 4

10 MINS

4 duck legs, skin on

4 tbsp korma curry paste

400ml tin of reduced-fat coconut milk

200g peeled and cored fresh pineapple, cut into chunks

3 tbsp dark soy sauce

1 red chilli, finely chopped, plus extra to garnish

Duck legs paired with a sweet and delicately spiced curry is about to become your new favourite. You can also use chicken legs here, if you prefer – both work so well with rice or noodles.

1 Feel free to skip this step, but I recommend searing the duck skin first in a hot pan without oil for 1–2 minutes, just to crisp up the skin.

2 Add the duck legs to the slow cooker with all the other ingredients and some salt and pepper and cook on high for 3 hours or low for 5–6 hours. If the sauce is looking a little thin, add 1 tablespoon of cornflour mixed with 1 tablespoon of water to thicken it up.

3 Once cooked, keep the duck legs whole or shred the meat off the bone. If you like crispy skin, then serve this as a garnish, if not, discard it. Scatter over extra chopped chilli and serve.

SERVING NOTE:
This works well on a bed of rice and garnished with coriander.

TIP: *If you don't have fresh pineapple, tinned pineapple chunks will work!*

PROTEIN: 72g | **CARBS:** 12g | **FAT:** 37g

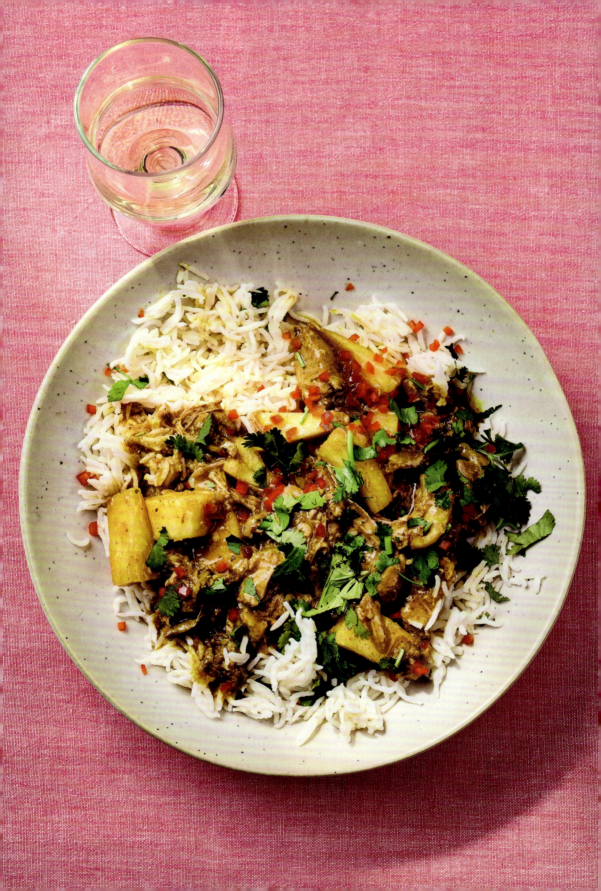

PORK SHOULDER THAI GREEN CURRY

424 CALORIES

SERVES 4

5 MINS

Pork shoulder in this simple curry with just five easy flavourings is rich and delicious; the meat becomes unbelievably tender in the slow cooker.

800g boneless pork shoulder, cut into chunks

200g mangetout

150g Thai green curry paste

400ml tin of reduced-fat coconut milk

2 tsp fish sauce

4 makrut lime leaves

1 Add all the ingredients to the slow cooker with 100ml of boiling water or chicken stock. Cook on high for 4 hours or low for 8 hours until the meat is completely tender.

2 Serve immediately.

SERVING NOTE:
Rice and lime wedges work best here. You could even add more veggies in, like baby corn and green beans.

TIP: *Cornflour is your saviour to thicken a sauce, if in doubt, add a tablespoon of cornflour mixed with a tablespoon of water at the end and stir it through.*

PROTEIN: 47g | **CARBS:** 9g | **FAT:** 21g

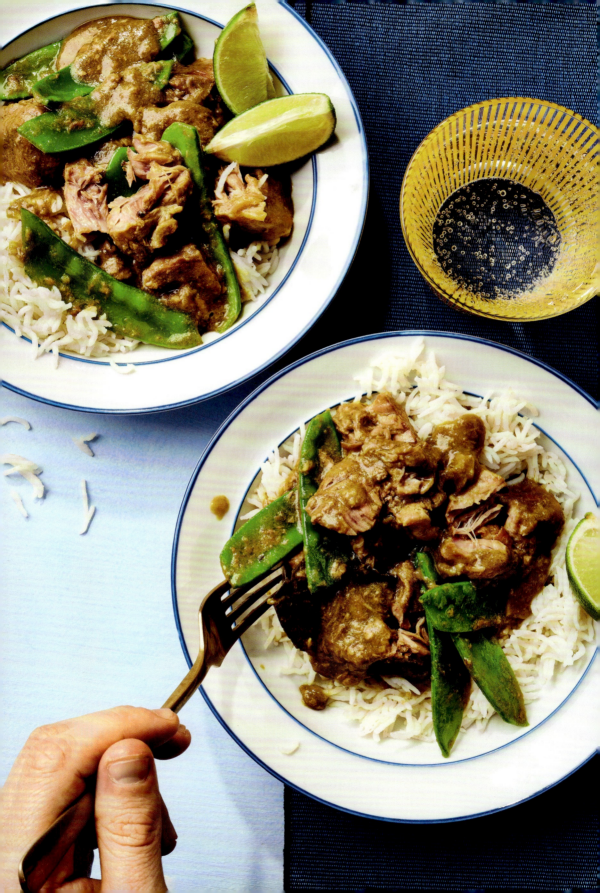

BEEF BRISKET MADRAS

395 CALORIES

SERVES 4

10 MINS

Much better than your local takeaway, and no long list of spices – just six ingredients. This curry is rich and full of warming flavours and is ideal served with rice or even potatoes.

600g beef brisket, unrolled

100g Madras spice paste

400g tin of chopped tomatoes

400ml tin of reduced-fat coconut milk

1 beef stock pot

1 tbsp garlic and ginger paste

1 Season the brisket while you heat a little oil in a large frying pan over a medium heat. Sear the brisket on all sides.

2 Transfer to the slow cooker with all the other ingredients and add 200ml of boiling water. Cook on high for 4 hours or low for 8 hours until the beef is soft.

3 Shred the meat using two forks in the pot, or, if you prefer, carefully remove the brisket from the sauce to a plate to do this, then return the beef to the slow cooker and stir to coat the meat.

4 Serve hot with rice or potatoes, if liked.

TIP: *Leftovers work perfectly in tacos or wraps.*

PROTEIN: 34g | **CARBS:** 11g | **FAT:** 24g

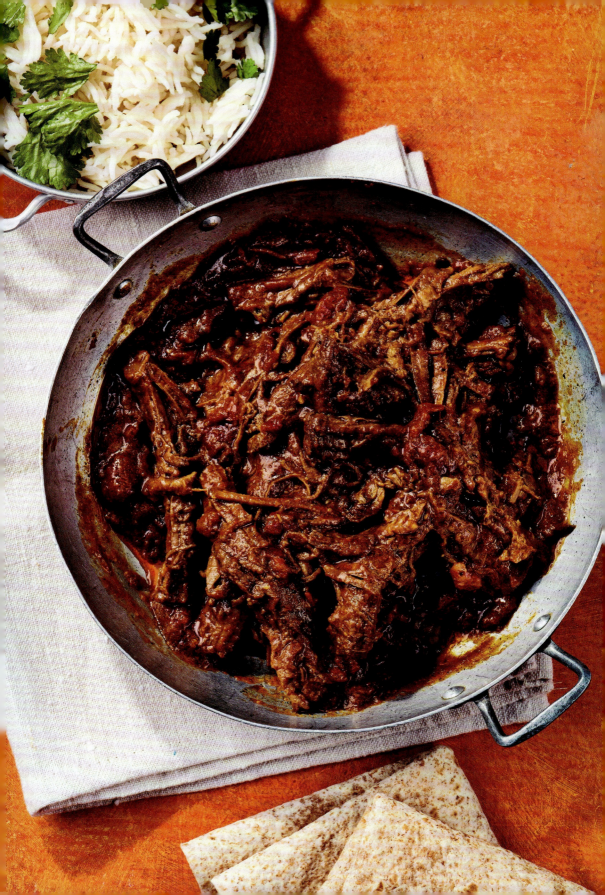

COMFORT
FOOD

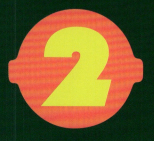

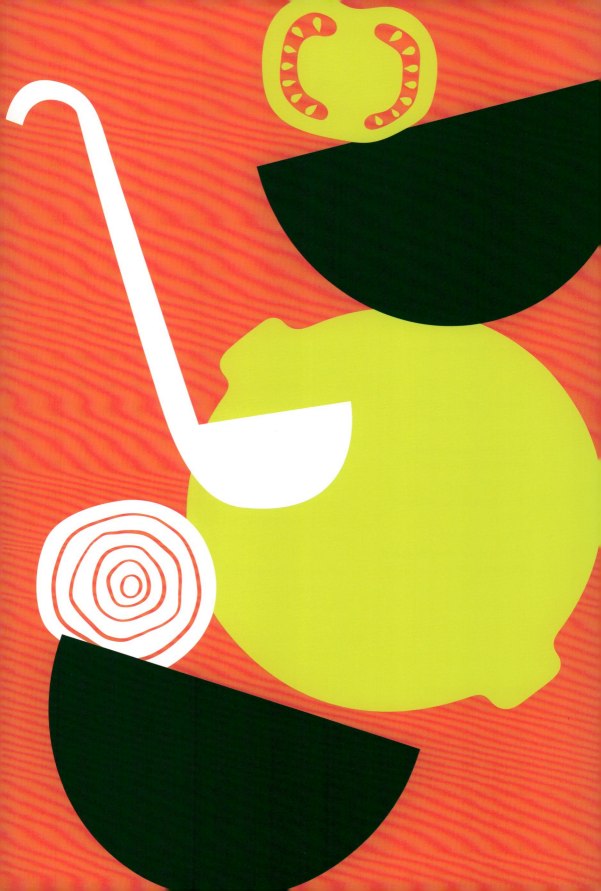

CHICKEN & BACON PIE

618 CALORIES

SERVES 6

15 MINS   (FILLING ONLY)

1 whole chicken, cut into 4 pieces (or 2 legs and 2 breasts)

12 smoked streaky bacon rashers, finely chopped

1 onion, finely diced

2 tbsp finely chopped fresh parsley

1 tbsp Dijon mustard

1 x 375g sheet of ready-rolled puff pastry, cut to fit using the slow cooker lid

SERVING NOTE:
Perfect with mash and peas!

TIP: *If you've got leftover cooked chicken, you could use this and skip step 1, going straight to step 2, adding the water or stock in then.*

Nothing screams comfort like a homemade pie, and this one could not be any easier.

1   Add the chicken pieces to the slow cooker, season with salt and pepper, then cover with 350ml of boiling water or chicken stock. Cook on high for 3 hours, or until the chicken is completely tender. Remove from the water to a plate and shred the meat using two forks, discarding the skin and bones. Set aside.

2   Add the bacon and onion to the slow cooker. Combine a couple of tablespoons of the water with 1 tablespoon of cornflour and add to the slow cooker, stirring it in. Cook on high for 1 hour until the bacon is cooked and the mixture has thickened to a coating consistency.

3   Return the shredded chicken to the slow cooker and add the parsley and Dijon mustard with some salt and pepper. Mix well and cook on high for 15 minutes to warm through.

4   Preheat the oven to 200°C. If your slow cooker dish is not ovenproof, decant the mixture into a baking dish. Add the puff pastry to the top of your pie (glazing it with egg, if preferred), then bake the pie for 15–20 minutes, or until the pastry is puffed and golden.

5   Serve immediately.

PROTEIN: 57g | **CARBS:** 26g | **FAT:** 32g

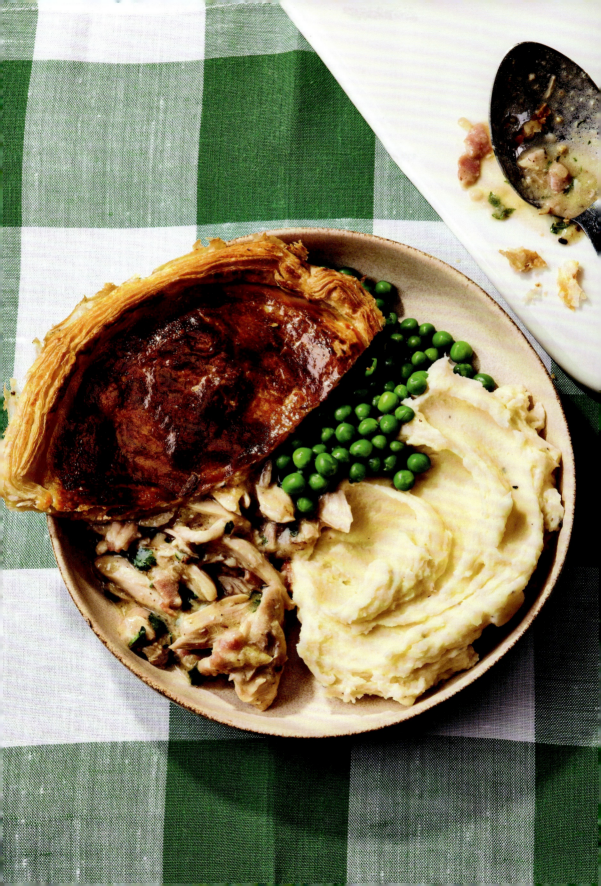

TARTIFLETTE

432 CALORIES

SERVES 6

15 MINS

An alpine classic with smoky bacon, lots of cheese and potatoes – what more could you want? Now this is a really hearty dish, so you'll definitely want to serve with a salad.

1kg Charlotte potatoes (or any waxy variety), cut into 5mm slices

1 onion, thinly sliced

200g smoked bacon lardons

50ml dry white wine

200ml single cream

1 x 250g whole Camembert cheese (or Reblochon, if you can find it)

1 Grease your slow cooker dish with butter or oil, then add in the potatoes, onion and lardons. Pour over the wine and cream, then move the mixture around until it is as flat as possible. Top the mixture with the whole Camembert, or slice it and lay the slices over the top of the dish to cover. Cook on high for 4 hours or low for 8 hours.

2 Once the potatoes are soft, place the slow cooker dish (make sure it's ovenproof) under a hot grill until the tartiflette bubbles and turns golden. Serve hot.

TIP: *If hosting a crowd with a roast dinner, this would make a great side rather than a main.*

PROTEIN: 14g | **CARBS:** 35g | **FAT:** 24g

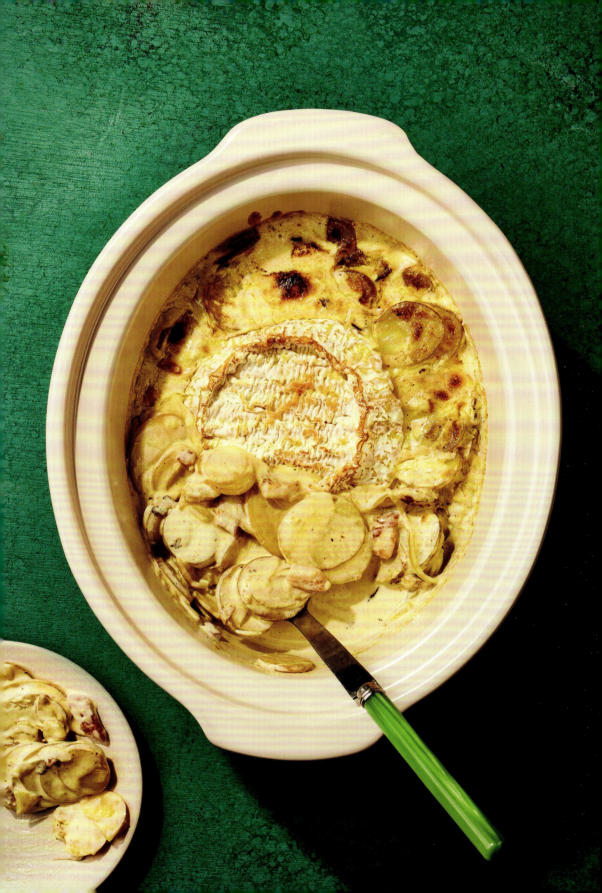

LAMB & CHICKPEA STEW WITH COUSCOUS

555 CALORIES

SERVES 4

10 MINS

This tagine-inspired stew is a firm favourite; the lamb is so tender and really packs some flavour from the delicious ras el hanout. You can't easily swap in other spices here as ras el hanout is made up of loads of spices – it's worth buying some to make this though!

600g boneless lamb shoulder or neck, cut into large chunks

1 onion, finely diced

2 tsp ras el hanout

1 tbsp tomato purée

400g tin of chickpeas, drained and rinsed

200g couscous

1 In a large frying pan, quickly sear the lamb in a little oil over a medium heat until sealed and golden before transferring to the slow cooker. You can skip this step, if you prefer, and just add the lamb straight to the slow cooker.

2 Add in all the other ingredients, except the couscous, along with 200ml of boiling water or chicken or lamb stock. Cook on high for 4 hours or low for 8 hours until the lamb is completely tender.

3 Add 1 tablespoon of cornflour mixed with 1 tablespoon of water to the slow cooker. Continue to cook for 30 minutes or until the mixture has thickened.

4 Meanwhile, add the couscous to a heatproof bowl and pour in enough boiling water to cover. Cover and leave for 10 minutes until the couscous has absorbed all the liquid and is soft. Fluff up with a fork and serve alongside the stew, scattered with chopped fresh coriander or parsley, if you like.

SERVING NOTE:
Pomegranate seeds scattered over the couscous add a lovely extra texture.

PROTEIN: 41g | **CARBS:** 54g | **FAT:** 18g

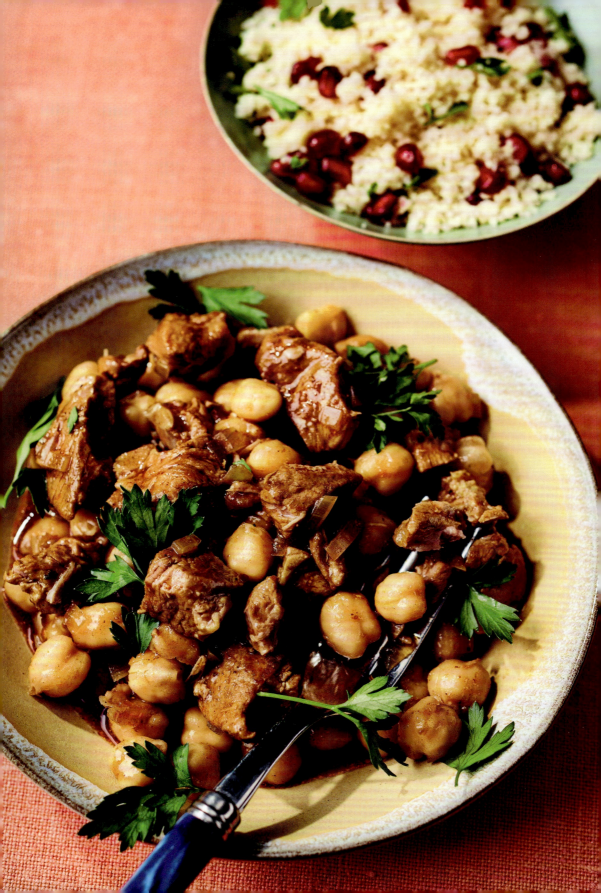

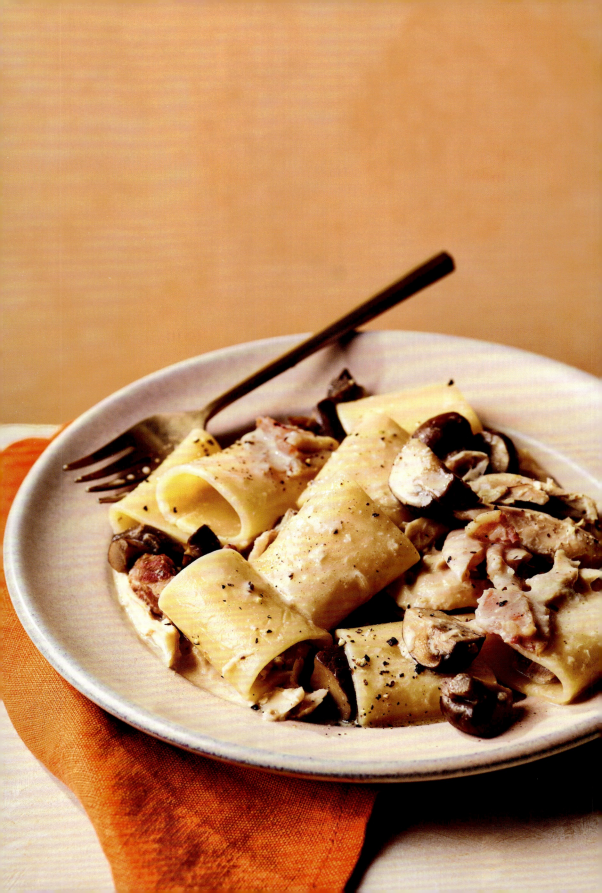

CREAMY CHICKEN PASTA WITH MUSHROOMS & BACON

784 CALORIES

SERVES 4

10 MINS   **(WITHOUT PASTA)**

1 whole chicken, cut into 8 pieces (or 2 legs and 2 breasts)

1 garlic bulb, peeled and cloves left whole

8 smoked streaky bacon rashers, chopped

250g chestnut mushrooms, quartered

50ml double cream

500g cooked pasta

I make this every week in the winter, even just for the two of us, and leave out the pasta so we can make different meals out of it. It's an easy one to make and freeze in batches, too.

1   Add all the ingredients, except the cream and pasta, to the slow cooker. Add 400ml of boiling water or chicken stock along with a pinch of salt and pepper. Cook on high for 4 hours or low for 8 hours until the chicken is completely tender.

2   Once cooked, you can leave the chicken on the bone and grill the pieces until golden, but I like to discard the skin and shred the meat into the sauce instead.

3   Use a spoon to squash the cooked garlic cloves and stir them into the sauce. Return the chicken to the pot and stir through the double cream.

4   Stir the sauce through the cooked pasta, season with pepper and serve.

TIP: *You could swap in mashed potato instead of the pasta, and serve the sauce alongside.*

PROTEIN: 85g | **CARBS:** 42g | **FAT:** 29g

BRAISED BEAN STEW

543 CALORIES

SERVES 4

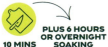 **PLUS 6 HOURS OR OVERNIGHT SOAKING**

10 MINS

 V

A vegan winter warmer, this is the easiest and most delicious bean stew. This hearty dish is the perfect comfort food, as you can throw in any type of beans you fancy here – the more the merrier! It's the ultimate one-pot meal that's perfect for cosy nights in.

500g dried beans, such as borlotti, pinto or cannellini

1 onion, thinly sliced

3 garlic cloves, peeled

400g tin of chopped tomatoes

500g Maris Piper potatoes, peeled and cut into small dice

1 tsp dried thyme or picked fresh thyme leaves, plus extra to garnish

1 Soak the beans in a bowl of cold water, ideally overnight or for at least 6 hours, to rehydrate.

2 Once soaked, drain the beans and add with all the ingredients to the slow cooker with 500ml of boiling water or stock. Cook on high for 3 hours or low for 6 hours until the beans and potatoes are completely soft.

3 Garnish with extra fresh thyme leaves if you have some, season with pepper and serve.

SERVING NOTE:
Buttered crusty bread is great for soaking up those delicious juices.

PROTEIN: 30g | **CARBS:** 98g | **FAT:** 2g

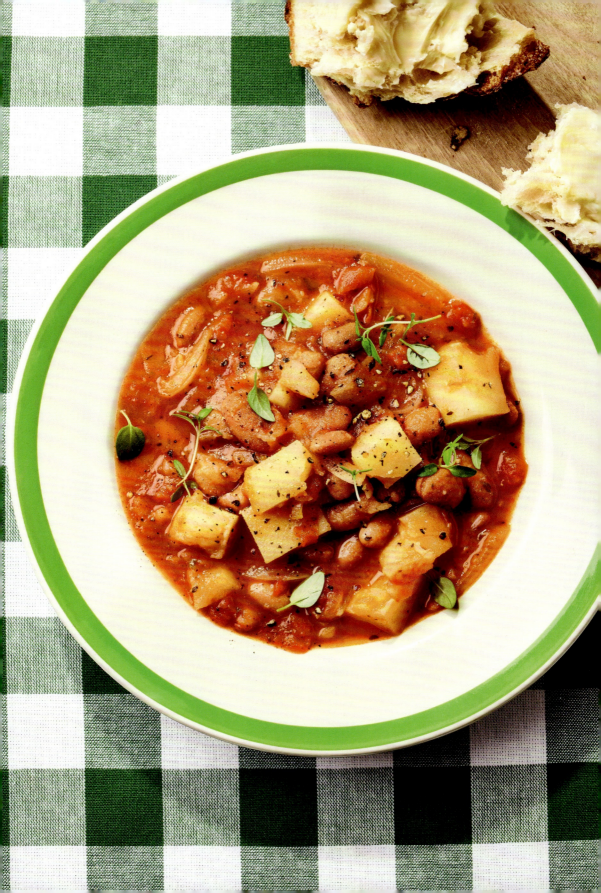

WINTER SAUSAGE MEATBALLS & CREAM

323 CALORIES

SERVES 4

10 MINS

On a cold day, this is perfection served with some nice crusty bread and another side of your choice – it's a very flexible dish that you can also enjoy with pasta or some gorgeous buttery colcannon or mash with green veg.

8–10 reduced-fat pork sausages

4 garlic cloves, crushed

3 tbsp Dijon mustard

1 tsp dried thyme

100ml double cream

2 handfuls of baby spinach leaves

1 Squeeze the sausage meat from the skins, then use wet hands to form it into 20 or so small meatballs.

2 Heat 1 tablespoon of oil in a frying pan, season the meatballs with salt and pepper and cook over a high heat for 1 minute to seal, turning regularly. This ensures they will stick together when cooked in the slow cooker.

3 Add the meatballs to the slow cooker with the garlic, mustard, thyme and 200ml of boiling water or chicken stock and let it do its thing on high for 3–4 hours or low for 7–8 hours.

4 Once cooked, stir in the cream and the spinach to wilt. If the sauce looks thin, add 1 tablespoon of cornflour mixed with a little water to thicken it. Serve and enjoy!

SERVING NOTE:
Peas and mash with spring onion stirred through works a dream here.

PROTEIN: 16g | **CARBS:** 14g | **FAT:** 23g

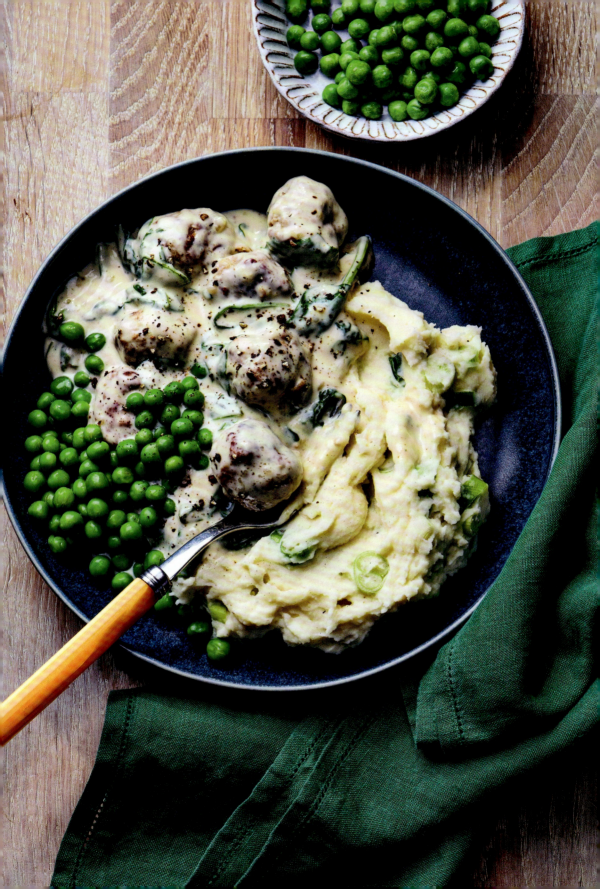

SIMPLE STEAK DIANE

257 CALORIES

SERVES 4

10 MINS

You can leave the steaks whole or cut them into chunks, but whatever you decide, this is a mouthwatering, gorgeous date-night dish. Buttery, creamy and with a dash of brandy or whiskey, this goes well with some simple mash and greens.

600g beef steaks, whole or cut into chunks

2 tbsp Dijon mustard

1 shot of brandy or whiskey

3 tbsp Worcestershire sauce

2 sprigs of fresh thyme

2 tbsp half-fat crème fraîche

1 Season and pan-fry the whole steaks or beef chunks for 1 minute on each side in a hot pan to sear, then melt 20g of half-fat butter and stir the steaks/chunks in the butter to coat.

2 Add the steaks/chunks to the slow cooker with 1–2 more knobs of butter and all the other ingredients, except the crème fraîche, adding in 200ml of boiling water or beef stock and a good amount of pepper. Cook on high for 3 hours or low for 5–6 hours. If the sauce is looking thin, add in 1 tablespoon of cornflour, first blended with a little of the sauce.

3 Once cooked, stir in the crème fraîche and serve with your sides of choice. Sensational.

SERVING NOTE:
Mash and green beans are my go-to here but air-fried chips would work equally well!

PROTEIN: 34g | **CARBS:** 4g | **FAT:** 10g

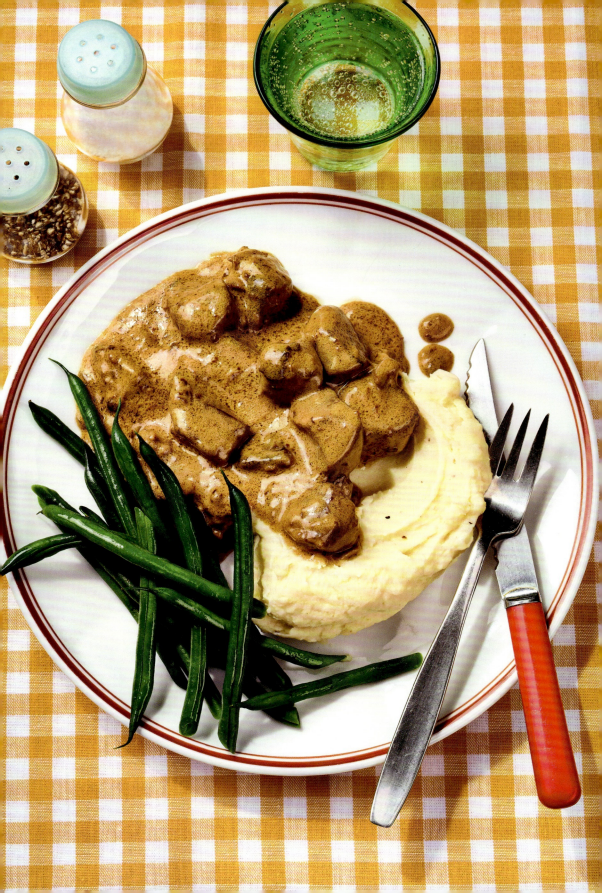

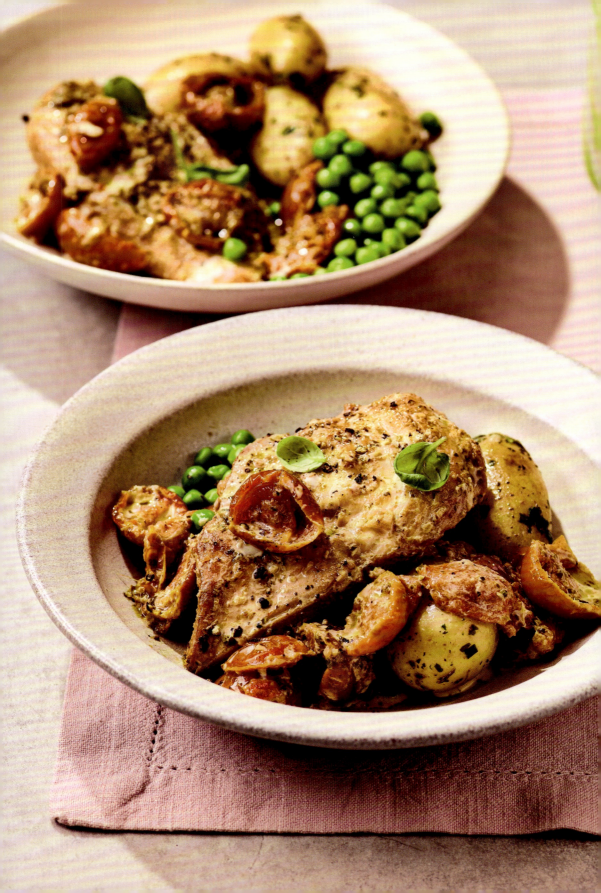

PESTO & SUNDRIED TOMATO CHICKEN

663 CALORIES

SERVES 4

10 MINS

Whether you choose red or green pesto, you'll be amazed at how something so simple can taste so delicious. This Italian-inspired dish pairs beautifully with a variety of sides and it's sure to become a favourite for any pesto lover.

4 chicken breasts, whole

180g jar of green pesto

200g sundried tomatoes

3 garlic cloves, crushed

2 tbsp half-fat crème fraîche

2 handfuls of fresh basil leaves, plus extra to garnish

1 If you like, slightly flatten the chicken breasts with a rolling pin and pan-fry them in 1 tablepoon of oil on each side for 1 minute. You can totally skip this step, though, if you prefer, as it cooks perfectly fine without.

2 Add all the ingredients to the slow cooker, apart from the crème fraîche and basil, adding 150ml of boiling water and 2 tablespoons of cornflour (mixed with a little water first), then cook on high for 3 hours or low for 5–6 hours.

3 Once cooked, remove the chicken breasts to serving plates. Stir the crème fraîche and basil into the sauce to combine, season with salt and pepper and then pour over the chicken. Garnish with more basil leaves and serve with your sides of choice.

SERVING NOTE:
A match made in heaven would be buttery new potatoes and peas.

PROTEIN: 40g | **CARBS:** 7g | **FAT:** 52g

CHEESY JALAPEÑO MINCE

304 CALORIES

SERVES 6

5 MINS   **(WITHOUT CHEESE)**

I am obsessed with doing tacos like this – it's a great way to use mince differently. If you like a spicy beef taco that might make your eyes water ever so slightly, this is for you. You can skip the jalapeños if you want a milder version. I normally stuff the mince into tortillas, but you could also serve this as a rice bowl.

500g lean beef mince

340g red enchilada sauce

2 onions, finely chopped

1 tbsp mild curry powder

4 fresh jalapeños, sliced

250g reduced-fat Cheddar cheese, grated

1 Add the beef mince, the enchilada sauce, the onions, the curry powder and 1 sliced jalapeño to the slow cooker with some salt and pepper. Cook on high for 4 hours or low for 7–8 hours.

2 Serve the mince mixture with the remaining sliced jalapeños and grated cheese scattered on top.

3 However, I suggest making tacos: place 12 mini tortillas on a large baking tray (or two) and then cover one half of each tortilla with the cheese, top with the mince and jalapeños and then fold in half and bake in the oven at 200°C for 7–8 minutes, or until the tacos are golden and the cheese has melted. You can also do this in the air fryer but you might have to do it in batches. Serve immediately with some roughly chopped coriander. These are mind-bogglingly good!

SERVING NOTE:
If making rice bowls, top some cooked rice with the mince mix, then sprinkle over the cheese and remaining sliced jalapeño.

PROTEIN: 30g | **CARBS:** 9g | **FAT:** 16g

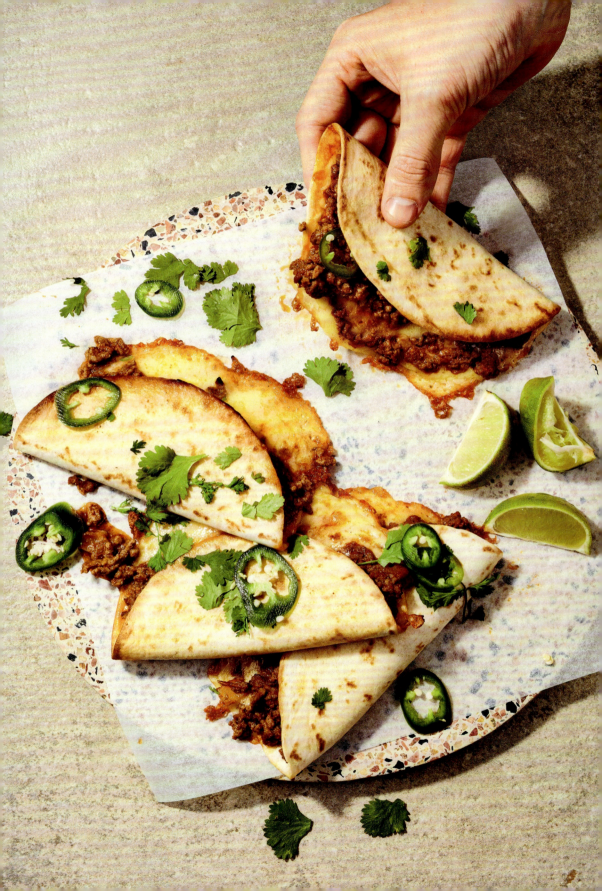

BEEF & BACON HOTPOT

458 CALORIES

SERVES 6

15 MINS

Hotpots in any form are the perfect winter warmer, and this really is a hug in a pot. I suggest using beef stock with a splash of red wine here, if you have some to hand – or forgo the wine and just use beef stock.

1kg braising steak, diced

8 smoked streaky bacon rashers, roughly chopped

3 sprigs of fresh rosemary or thyme, plus extra leaves to garnish

2 onions, chopped

500ml beef stock

500g potatoes, thinly sliced (leave the skin on)

1 Brown the beef in a hot frying pan in 1 tablespoon of oil for 2 minutes, then add the bacon and cook everything for another few minutes.

2 Once the beef is seared and the bacon golden, add the beef and bacon and all the other ingredients, apart from the potatoes, to the slow cooker and season well with salt and pepper. Cook on high for 3–4 hours or low for 6–7 hours.

3 For the last hour and a half of cooking, add 2 heaped tablespoons of cornflour blended with 2 tablespoons of water to the slow cooker and mix in. Then layer the thinly sliced potatoes on top, season with black pepper and allow them to cook in the slow cooker.

4 Once the last hour and a half is up, brush the top of the potatoes with 1 tablespoon of oil and place the ovenproof slow cooker pot under a hot grill for 10–15 minutes, or until the potatoes start to go golden. Serve immediately, garnished with extra rosemary or thyme leaves.

TIP: *Slice the potatoes as thinly as you can!*

PROTEIN: 45g | **CARBS:** 27g | **FAT:** 19g

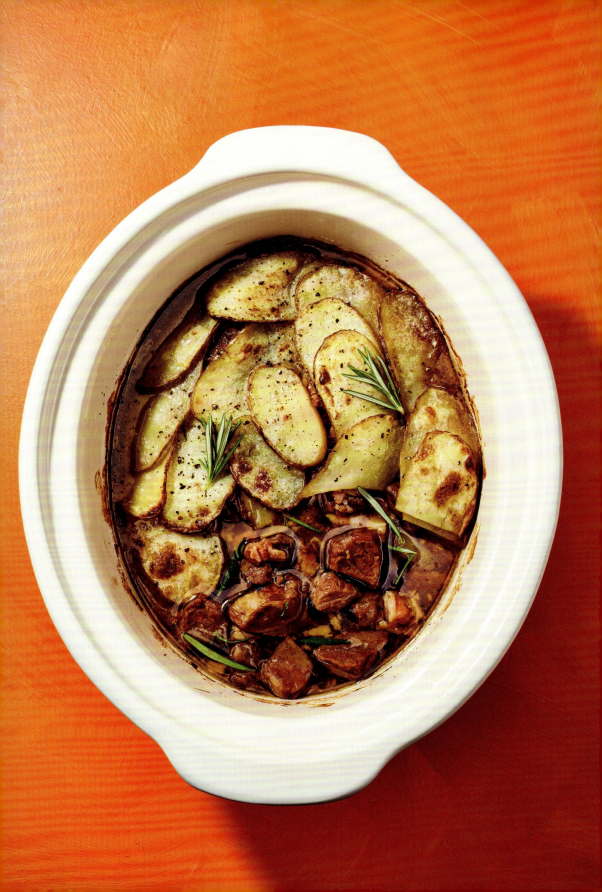

CREAMY PORK SAUSAGE PASTA

382 CALORIES

SERVES 6

10 MINS

I believe it is totally impossible to go wrong with a pork sausage dish. This moreishly rich sausage pasta dish is beyond simple. I use pesto because it packs a bigger punch, but feel free to use tomato purée or passata.

12 reduced-fat pork sausages

1 onion, finely chopped

3 tbsp tomato pesto (I love sundried)

550g cooked penne pasta

handful of fresh basil leaves

2 tbsp half-fat crème fraîche

1 Cut up the sausages with scissors or a sharp knife, discard the skins (you can leave on, if you like, though) and briefly pan-fry for 1–2 minutes, until browned.

2 Add the sausage pieces to the slow cooker with the onion, pesto and 50ml of boiling water or chicken stock and season with salt and pepper. Cook on high for 3–4 hours or low for 7–8 hours.

3 Once cooked, stir in the cooked pasta, basil leaves and crème fraîche, season with black pepper and serve.

PROTEIN: 23g | **CARBS:** 47g | **FAT:** 11g

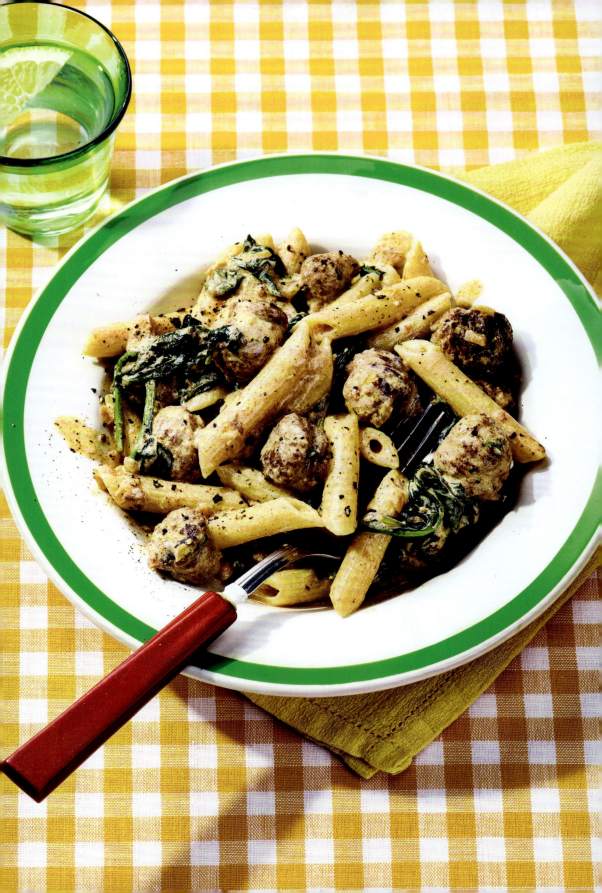

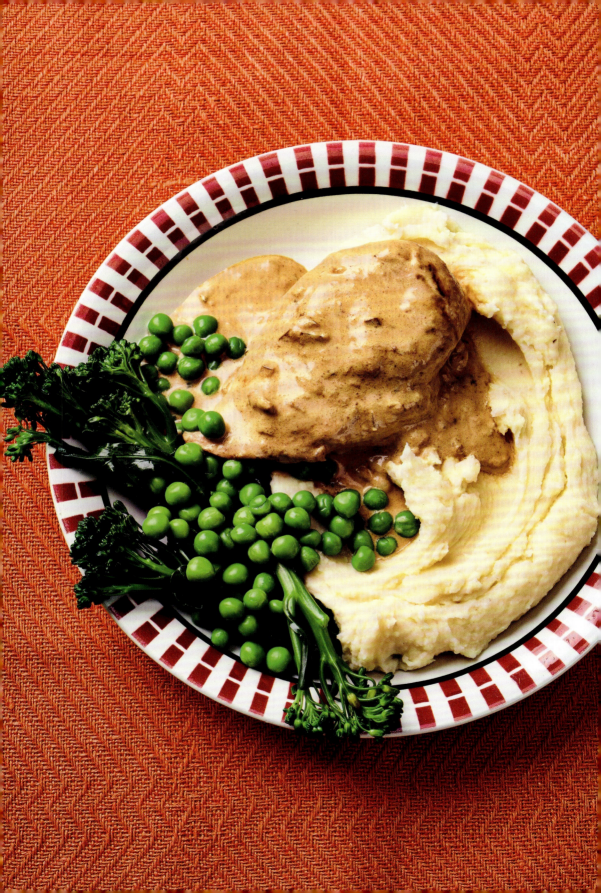

CREAMY WHITE WINE CHICKEN

223 CALORIES

SERVES 4

10 MINS

Chicken, cream and white wine, I don't even need to try to sell you this recipe as it is just divine and beyond simple to make. It's ideal for both busy weeknights and special occasions.

4 chicken breasts, whole

100ml white wine

2 tbsp Dijon mustard

1 onion, finely diced

3 garlic cloves, crushed

3 tbsp half-fat crème fraîche

1 In a hot frying pan, heat/melt a little oil or butter and cook the chicken breasts for 1–2 minutes on each side until sealed all over.

2 Add the chicken and all the buttery goodness from the pan to the slow cooker with all the other ingredients, except the crème fraîche. Add 50ml of boiling water or chicken stock.

3 Cook on high for 4 hours or low for 7–8 hours, then stir in the crème fraîche.

SERVING NOTE:
Serve with some green veg, and this goes incredibly well with a creamy cheesy mash, too.

PROTEIN: 37g | **CARBS:** 4g | **FAT:** 4g

GARLIC BUTTER CHICKEN WITH BACON & SWEETCORN

552 CALORIES

SERVES 4

10 MINS

I tried something very similar to this dish in Florida and I knew that whatever way this was made I would suss out how to do it when I got home. And here we are. Garlic butter chicken is divine on its own, but add in crispy bacon and creamy corn and that's next level.

4 chicken breasts, whole

2 tbsp Cajun seasoning

2 x 340g tins of sweetcorn

4 tbsp shop-bought garlic butter (or see Tip)

6 smoked streaky bacon rashers

50ml double cream

1 Coat the chicken breasts in 1 tablespoon of the Cajun seasoning and some salt and pepper, then seal in a hot frying pan in 1 tablespoon of oil for 1 minute on each side.

2 Add the sealed chicken to the slow cooker with the sweetcorn, garlic butter and remaining Cajun seasoning. Cook on high for 4 hours or low for 7 hours.

3 When the chicken is cooked, air-fry or crisp the bacon in the oven, then slice it up and stir through the chicken mixture with the cream.

4 Serve with some green beans, if you like.

TIP: *You can make your own garlic butter by combining softened butter, crushed garlic and finely chopped fresh parsley.*

PROTEIN: 46g | **CARBS:** 18g | **FAT:** 32g

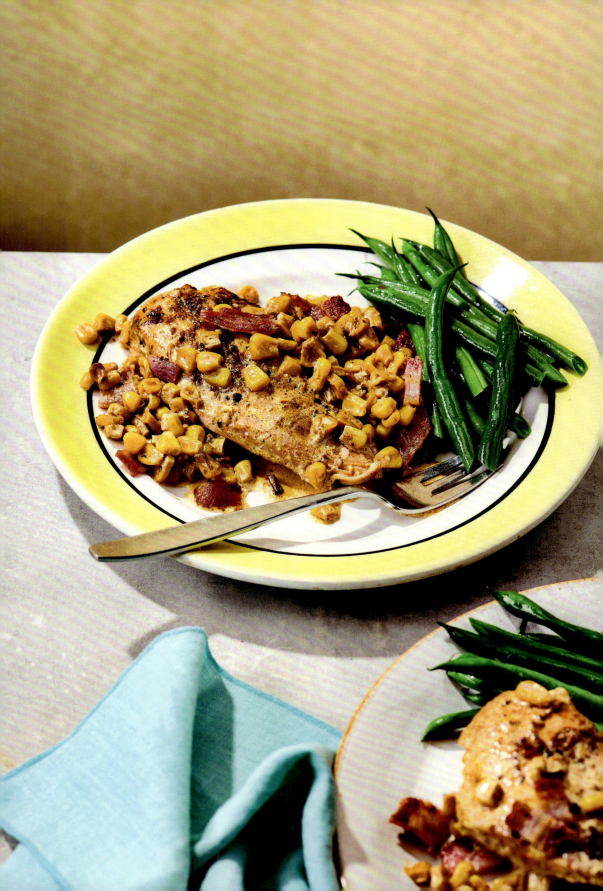

RICH PORK SAUSAGE & PORCINI RAGÙ

220 CALORIES

SERVES 4

10 MINS

A ragù features in all my slow cooker books, and this book is no exception. I get excited when I think about what I can turn a packet of sausages into, so I came up with this stripped-back sausage and mushroom ragù. It's delicious.

8 reduced-fat pork sausages

50g dried porcini mushrooms or 200g fresh chestnut mushrooms, thinly sliced

3 garlic cloves, thinly sliced

400g passata

1 rich beef stock pot

1 tsp fresh thyme leaves, plus extra to garnish

1　Squeeze the sausages from their skins, break up into small chunks and pan-fry in 1 tablespoon of oil over a medium heat until golden.

2　Add the sausage meat chunks to the slow cooker with all the other ingredients, then add 150ml of boiling water and season well with salt and pepper. Cook on high for 3–4 hours or low for 7–8 hours.

3　Serve.

SERVING NOTE:
Serve with cooked pasta stirred through (I like pacheri or tagliatelle) and some extra thyme leaves sprinkled on top to garnish.

PROTEIN: 16g | **CARBS:** 17g | **FAT:** 9g

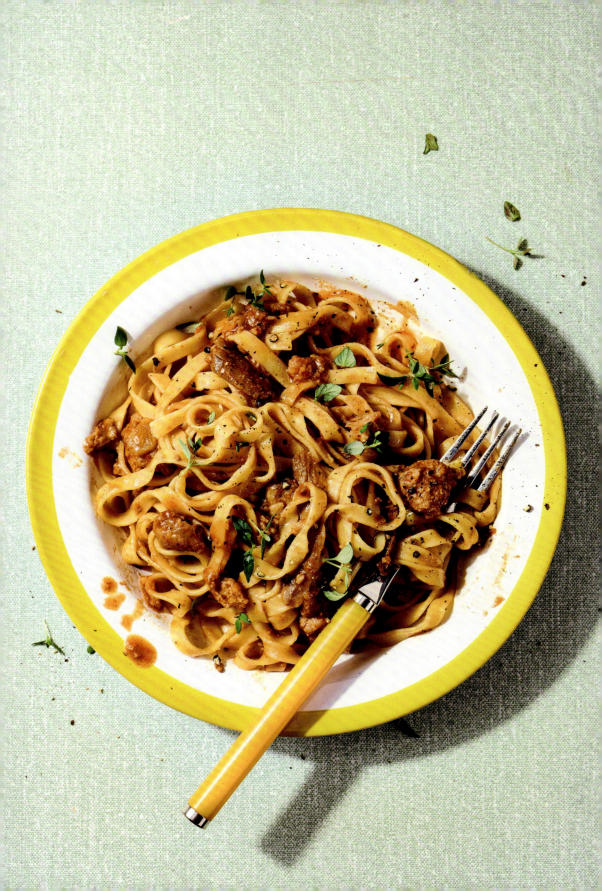

SOUPS, LUNCHES & LIGHTER MEALS

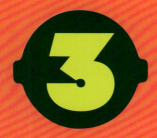

3

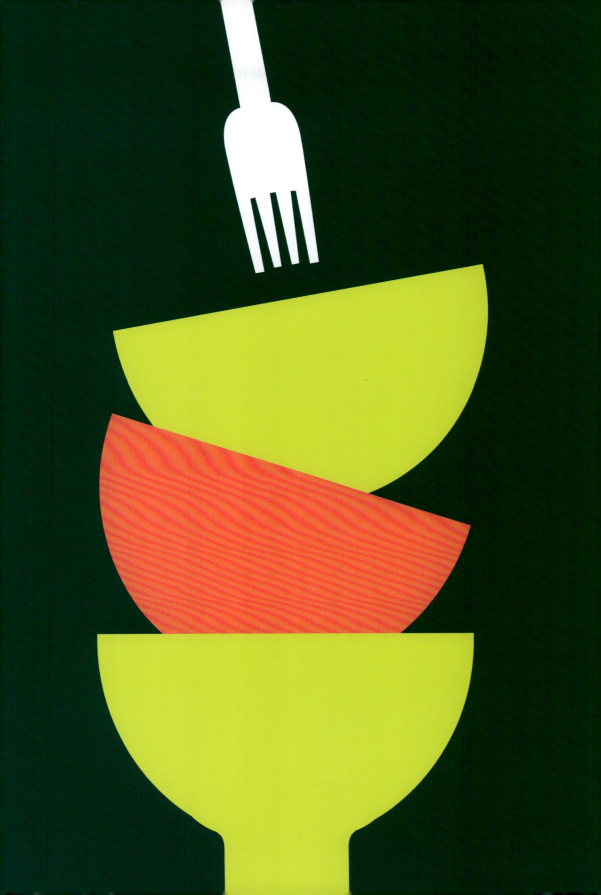

SPICED SWEET POTATO & HALLOUMI SOUP

349 CALORIES

SERVES 6

25 MINS

If halloumi is in a recipe, then I'm cooking it. It's such a versatile ingredient and I must easily eat a block a week. This recipe helps me maintain that consistent halloumi devouring.

1.2kg sweet potatoes, peeled and cut into small chunks

4 tbsp curry paste of your choice, or a few tbsp curry powder

1 onion, sliced

2 carrots, peeled and roughly chopped

3 garlic cloves, crushed

1 x 250g block of reduced-fat halloumi, sliced or cubed

1 Tip the sweet potato chunks onto a roasting tray and coat in the curry paste or powder. Roast in the air fryer for 10 minutes at 200°C or in the oven (at the same temperature) for 15 minutes.

2 Add to the slow cooker with all the other ingredients, except the halloumi. Add 1.2 litres of boiling water or stock, then cook on high for 3 hours or low for 6 hours. Once cooked, blitz in the slow cooker with a hand blender until smooth and season with salt and pepper.

3 Pan-fry or air-fry the halloumi until golden all over, then scatter the halloumi pieces over the soup in bowls to serve. Divine.

PROTEIN: 14g | **CARBS:** 46g | **FAT:** 10g

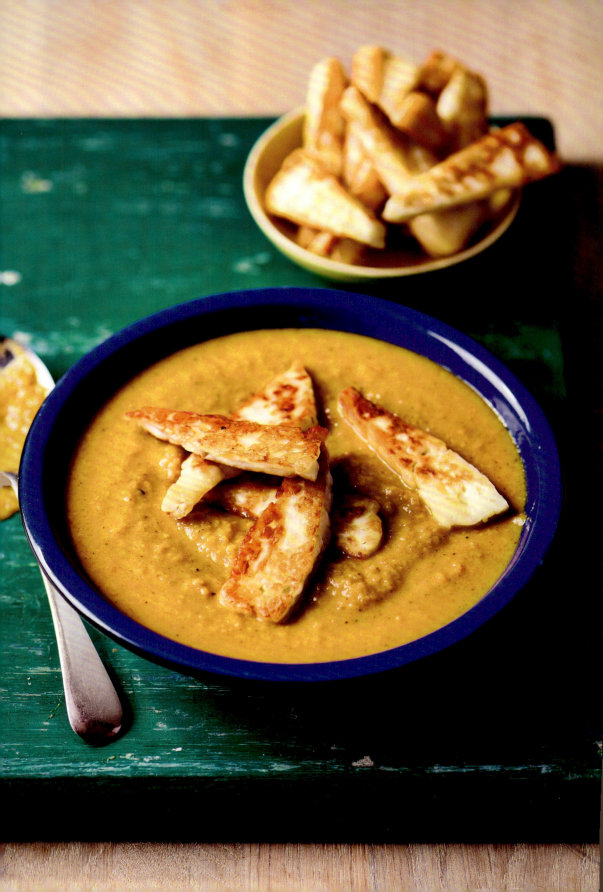

RED THAI CURRY SOUP

175 CALORIES

SERVES 4

5 MINS

This is the perfect recipe to put on on those cold winter mornings. Fragrant and warming with a fiery kick, if you made it in the morning it will be ready for your lunch!

4 tbsp red Thai curry paste

400ml tin of reduced-fat coconut milk

200g raw large peeled prawns (with tails left on), or boneless and skinless chicken thighs, sliced

2 red peppers, sliced

200g mangetout

chopped spring onions, to serve

1 Whisk together the curry paste and coconut milk until smooth. Add to the slow cooker with the prawns or chicken, sliced red peppers and 600ml of boiling water or chicken stock. Stir well and cook on high for 2 hours or low for 4 hours. Add the mangetout or broccoli halfway through.

2 Once cooked, divide among bowls and serve topped with chopped spring onions. Scatter over some finely chopped red chilli and chopped fresh coriander, if you like.

TIP: *You can throw in any veg here; Tenderstem broccoli, for example, would really bulk out the meal a bit more.*

PROTEIN: 12g | **CARBS:** 11g | **FAT:** 9g

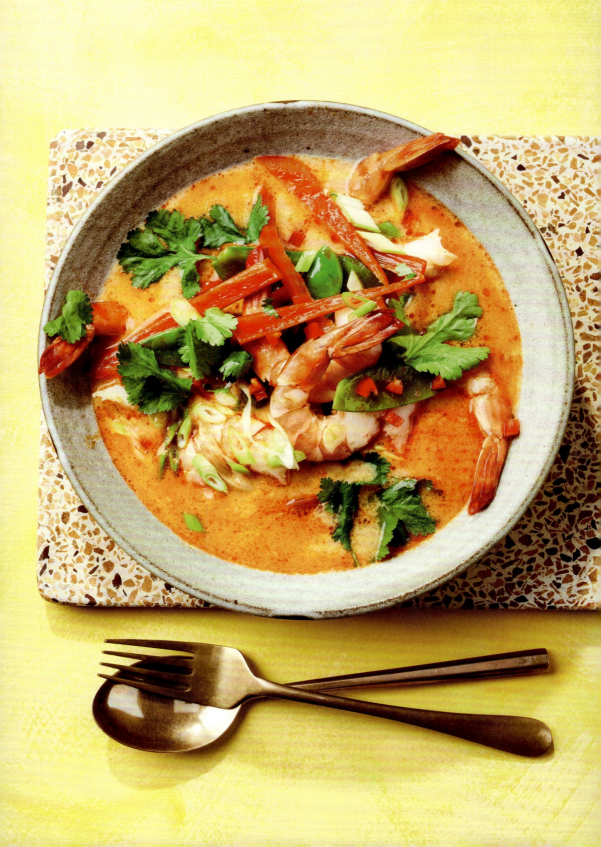

HAM HOCK & SPLIT PEA SOUP

278 CALORIES

SERVES 8

10 MINS

You get so much amazing flavour from a ham hock, it's a shame to waste it on a few portions. This recipe makes 8 servings, so there's plenty to store in the freezer.

400g dried yellow split peas, rinsed

1 onion, finely diced

2 carrots, peeled and diced

1 celery stick, diced

2 garlic cloves, crushed

400g cooked ham hock, shredded

1 Add all the ingredients, except the ham hock, to the slow cooker and cover with 1.5 litres of boiling water or chicken stock. Cook on high for 3–4 hours or low for 5–6 hours.

2 Stir the soup well, then blitz in the slow cooker with a hand blender if you prefer a smoother texture. Add the ham with a good pinch of salt and pepper.

3 Serve with lots of crusty bread and butter, if liked.

TIP: *Cooking a ham hock, gammon or small ham in the slow cooker really brings in lots of flavour, so if you can get your hands on one (800g bone-in or 600g boneless), it's worth it. Add it to the slow cooker with the split peas and just make sure to remove and shred before you blitz the soup.*

PROTEIN: 21g | **CARBS:** 32g | **FAT:** 8g

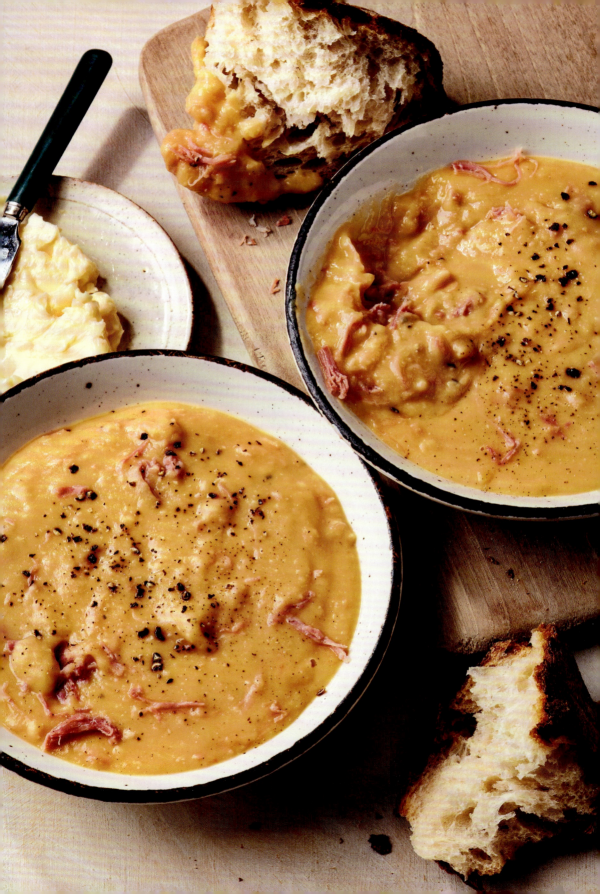

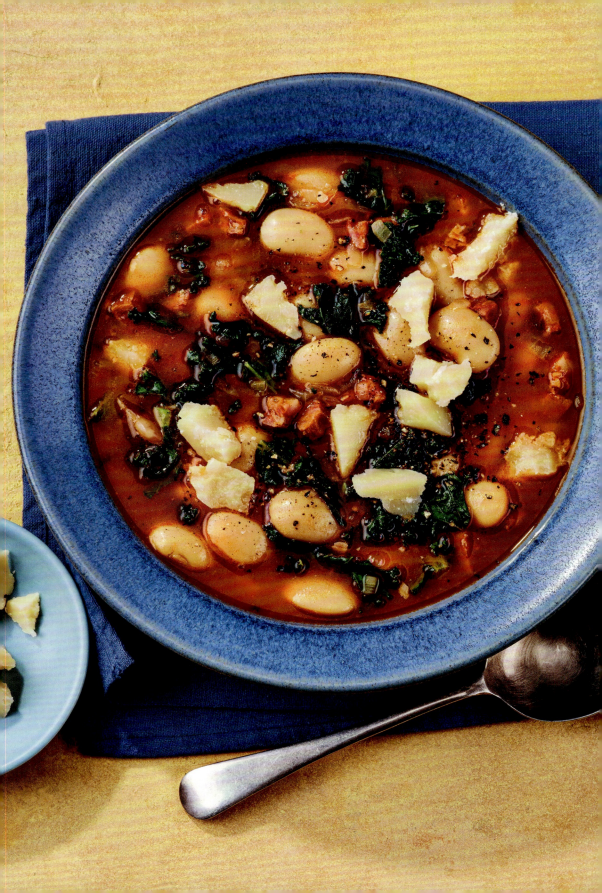

CHORIZO & BUTTER BEAN SOUP

336 CALORIES

SERVES 4

5 MINS

This soup will warm your soul. It's perfect for those chilly evenings when you crave something delicious and comforting. It's super easy to whip up and is bursting with bold, slightly spicy flavours.

1 onion, finely diced

2 garlic cloves, crushed

200g chorizo, finely diced

1 tbsp tomato purée

2 x 400g tins of butter beans, drained and rinsed

150g baby spinach leaves

1 Add all the ingredients, except the spinach, to the slow cooker with a good pinch of salt and pepper and 750ml of boiling water or chicken stock. Cook on high for 2 hours or low for 4 hours.

2 Check the seasoning, then serve in bowls, with the spinach added to gently wilt in the heat of the soup. You could also crumble or grate over some Parmesan cheese, if you like.

TIP: *Spinach or kale work equally well in this soup – kale gives an added texture, too.*

PROTEIN: 21g | **CARBS:** 20g | **FAT:** 17g

GINGER, PAK CHOI & PRAWN SOUP

312 CALORIES

SERVES 4

5 MINS

Get ready to fall in love with this Vietnamese-inspired soup. This is perfect for when you're feeling a little run-down and need some delicious wellness in a bowl. Fresh, punchy and oh so good.

600ml pho broth (you can use stock or bone broth, if unavailable)

large piece of fresh ginger, peeled and cut into 3–4 pieces

12–16 raw large peeled prawns (with tails left on)

250g rice noodles

4 pak choi, sliced in half, or into quarters if large

1 tbsp roughly chopped fresh coriander

1 Add the broth and ginger to the slow cooker and heat on high for 10–15 minutes.

2 Add the prawns, noodles and pak choi and cook on high for 1 hour, or until the prawns are pink and cooked through and the noodles are tender.

3 Divide between bowls, ensuring each bowl gets a good mix of prawns, noodles and pak choi. Top with the coriander and serve hot.

SERVING NOTE:
You could serve this with bean sprouts, lime wedges, fresh mint and chilli sauce to bulk this out.

PROTEIN: 19g | **CARBS:** 55g | **FAT:** 1g

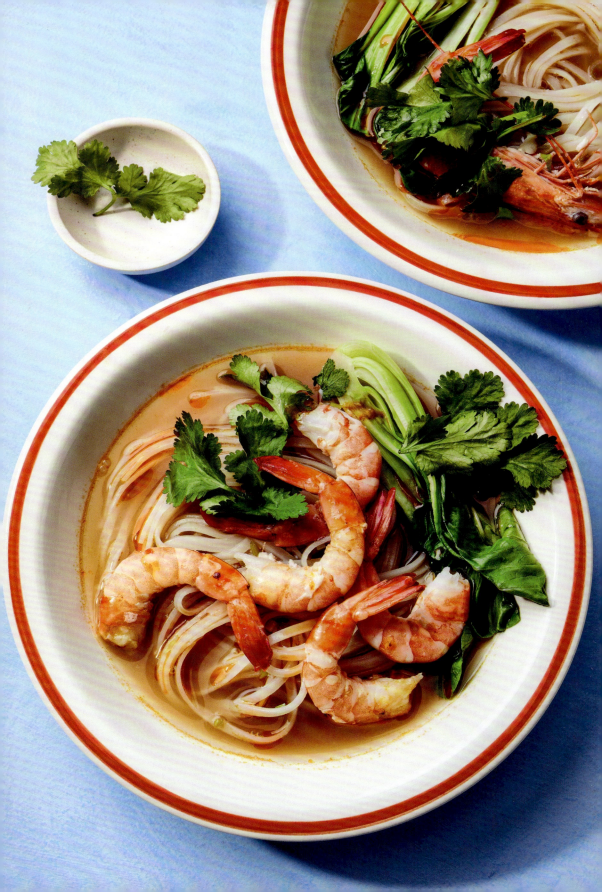

BROCCOLI, LEEK & STILTON SOUP

225 CALORIES

SERVES 6

10 MINS

It's no secret that cheese and veg work really well together and this cheesy veg soup is one you will come back to time and time again. Simple and very cost-effective, it's a favourite of mine.

2 heads of broccoli, cut into florets, keep the stalks for the garnish (optional)

1 large onion, sliced

4 garlic cloves, grated

2 leeks, sliced

120g Stilton cheese, crumbled, plus extra to garnish

100ml double cream

1 Add all the ingredients, apart from the broccoli stalks, cheese and cream to the slow cooker. Season generously with salt and pepper, then add 1 litre of boiling water or chicken stock. Cook on high for 3 hours or low for 6 hours.

2 Around 20 minutes before the soup is ready, if using the broccoli stalks, cut them into smaller pieces/batons, then toss with some oil, salt and pepper and roast on a baking tray in the oven at 200°C for 20 minutes, or in an air fryer for the same amount of time. (Or you can skip this step.)

3 Heads up: when you take the lid off the soup, it won't smell overly inviting – broccoli has that effect, but trust the process. Add the Stilton and cream and blitz in the slow cooker with a hand blender until smooth. Serve topped with more crumbled Stilton, and the roasted broccoli stalks, if using. Finish with an extra grind of pepper.

PROTEIN: 9g | **CARBS:** 7g | **FAT:** 17g

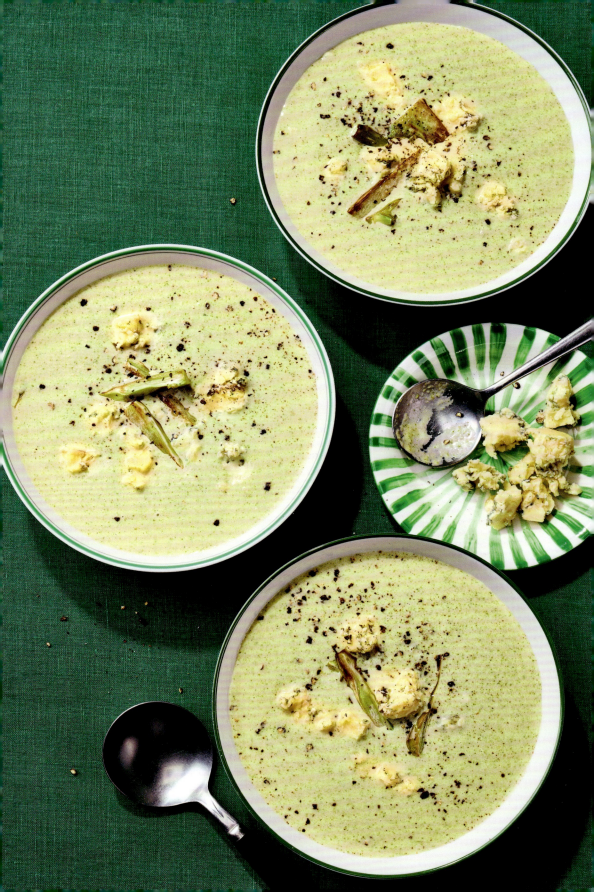

CREAMY CHICKEN & POTATO SOUP

448 CALORIES

SERVES 6

15 MINS

This is a comforting classic and a soup that my friend's mum made us when we were younger. It was different every time she made it, so it's definitely a throw whatever you want in each time kind of soup. Heavenly comfort in a bowl.

400g chicken breasts, whole

4 leeks, finely chopped

2 tbsp dried mixed Italian herbs

4 garlic cloves, grated or crushed

1kg potatoes, peeled and cut into chunks (I quarter them)

200ml double cream

1 Add the chicken, a good knob of butter, the leeks, dried herbs, garlic, potatoes and some salt and pepper to the slow cooker, along with 1 litre of boiling water or chicken stock. Cook on high for 3 hours or low for 6 hours.

2 Remove half the potatoes and the chicken to a plate and shred the chicken with two forks, then blitz the broth in the slow cooker using a hand blender until smooth.

3 Return the shredded chicken and potatoes to the blended broth before stirring through the double cream. You can stir in 1 tablespoon of cornflour mixed with 1 tablespoon water to thicken, if required. Serve in bowls with an extra grind of pepper on top.

SERVING NOTE:
Serve this with some crusty bread and butter.

PROTEIN: 29g | **CARBS:** 35g | **FAT:** 21g

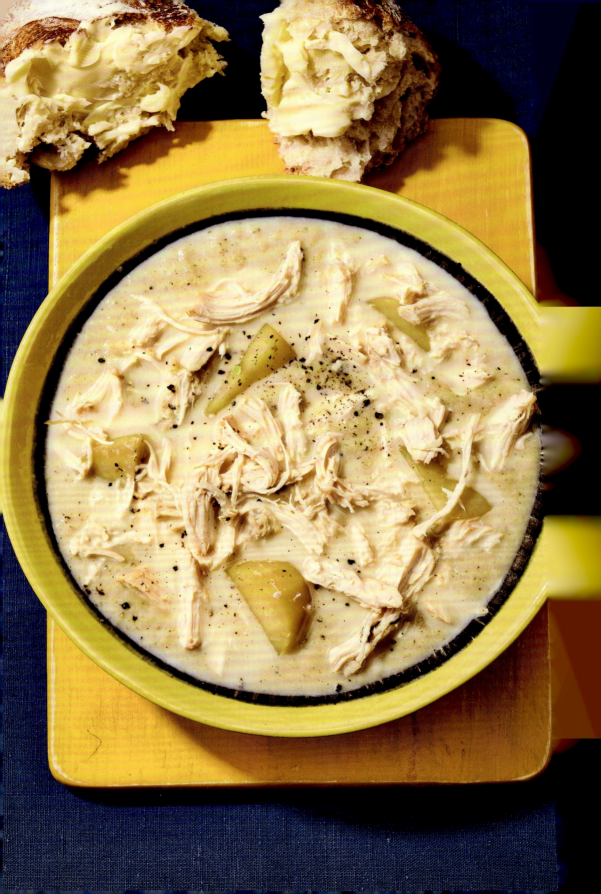

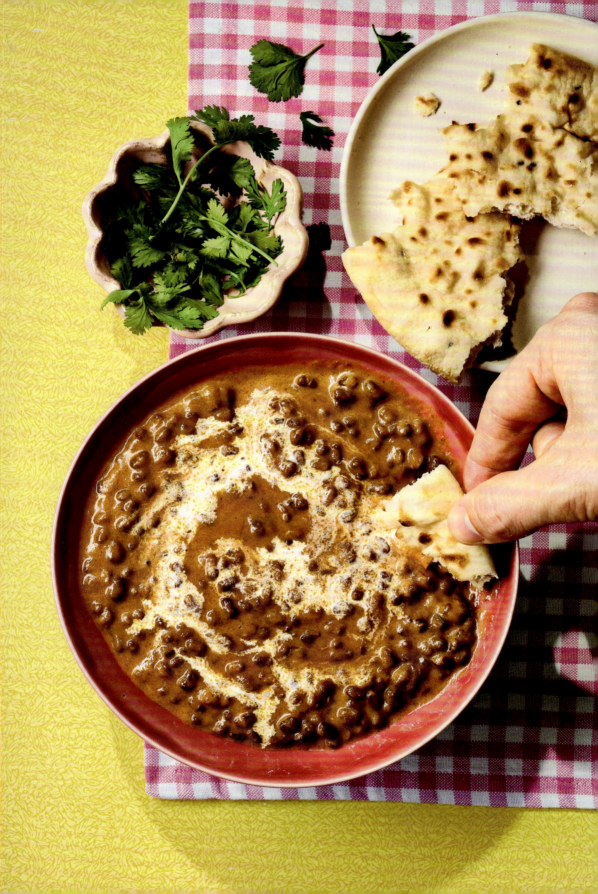

BLACK LENTIL DAHL

481 CALORIES

SERVES 4

10 MINS

This gorgeous black dahl is an alternative spin on one of my favourite midweek meals. I hadn't tried black dahls until having this in a London restaurant and it's now a firm favourite. Where have these been all my life? Feel free to add some cream in at the end.

250g dried whole black lentils

2 tbsp curry paste (I love korma with this one)

400g passata

4 garlic cloves, grated

100g half-fat butter

100ml double cream (optional)

1   Add all the ingredients to the slow cooker, apart from the cream, along with 900ml of boiling water or chicken stock and some salt and pepper.

2   Cook on high for 4 hours or low for 8 hours.

3   Stir in the cream, if using, season and enjoy.

SERVING NOTE:
Perfect with warm flatbreads for dunking in. You could also garnish the bowls of dahl with some fresh coriander leaves scattered over.

PROTEIN: 17g | **CARBS:** 36g | **FAT:** 28g

CHUNKY BACON, LEEK & POTATO SOUP

271 CALORIES

SERVES 6

10 MINS

Potato and leek soup is one of my favourite soups, so this stripped-back, non-blitzed version with bacon is all you need on a cold day – or any day, for that matter. The chicken stock really packs in that flavour, so don't swap it with water here.

8 smoked streaky bacon rashers

4 large potatoes, roughly chopped, skin on

3 leeks, sliced

2 tbsp dried mixed herbs

4 garlic cloves, grated

1.1 litres chicken stock

1 Cut up the bacon and briefly pan-fry in 1 tablespoon of oil over a medium heat until golden.

2 Add the bacon to the slow cooker with all the other ingredients and some salt and pepper. Cook on high for 2–3 hours or low for 5–6 hours.

3 Do not blitz, simply serve in bowls and enjoy. You can add some cream if you have some spare or that needs using. You could add a little chopped fresh dill as a garnish, too.

SERVING NOTE:
Serve this with some crusty bread and butter.

PROTEIN: 14g | **CARBS:** 30g | **FAT:** 10g

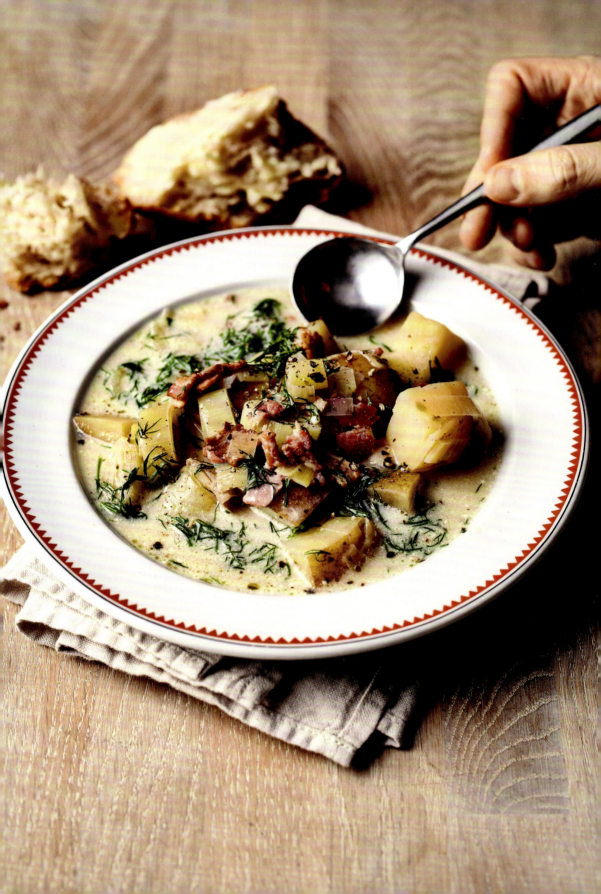

HARISSA & CHORIZO SHAKSHUKA

438 CALORIES

SERVES 4

10 MINS

This is PERFECT for hosting; if your family or guests have stayed over, here is a fuss-free way to wake them up with a kick. If this is more lunch-orientated than brunch, I would use curry paste instead of harissa.

200g chorizo, cut into cubes

3 x 400g tins of chopped tomatoes

1 tbsp harissa paste

1 shallot, finely chopped

handful of fresh parsley, chopped, plus extra to garnish

4 eggs

1   Add all the ingredients, except the eggs, to the slow cooker and season well with salt and pepper. Cook on high for 2–3 hours.

2   Stir through 100ml of boiling water, then create four wells or indents with a cup, breaking an egg into each well/indent as you go. Season the eggs with black pepper, then pop the lid back on and cook on high for a further 25 minutes – depending on your slow cooker, it may need more or less but keep an eye on it. Scatter over some extra chopped parsley, season with black pepper, then tuck in and enjoy.

TIP: *If you have one of those timer plugs, you could get this ready the night before and set it to turn on early in the morning, ready for breakfast.*

PROTEIN: 23g | **CARBS:** 13g | **FAT:** 22g

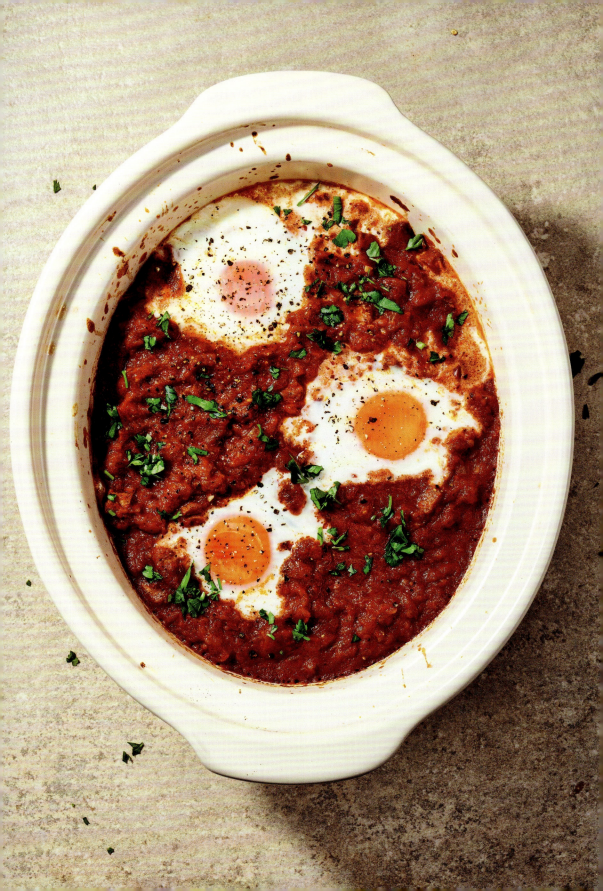

CURRIED LENTILS & LEEKS

SERVES 4

5 MINS

This is a dish that feels like pure heaven to me. It's such a gorgeous quick lunch of curried leeks with lentils to fill you up. Perfect for any time of the year, this is a comforting and nutritious option that will leave you feeling full and happy!

3 leeks, thickly sliced

2 tbsp curry paste of your choice, ideally with garlic

1 red chilli, sliced

1 tbsp tomato purée

300ml vegetable stock

200g pouch of cooked Puy lentils

1 Add all the ingredients to the slow cooker, except the lentils, adding in a good knob of butter or 1 tablespoon of oil and some salt and pepper. Cook on high for 3 hours or low for 6 hours.

2 Stir in the lentils in the last 15 minutes of the cooking time and leave to warm through.

3 Serve in bowls, garnished with coriander, if liked, and enjoy.

PROTEIN: 8g | **CARBS:** 16g | **FAT:** 6g

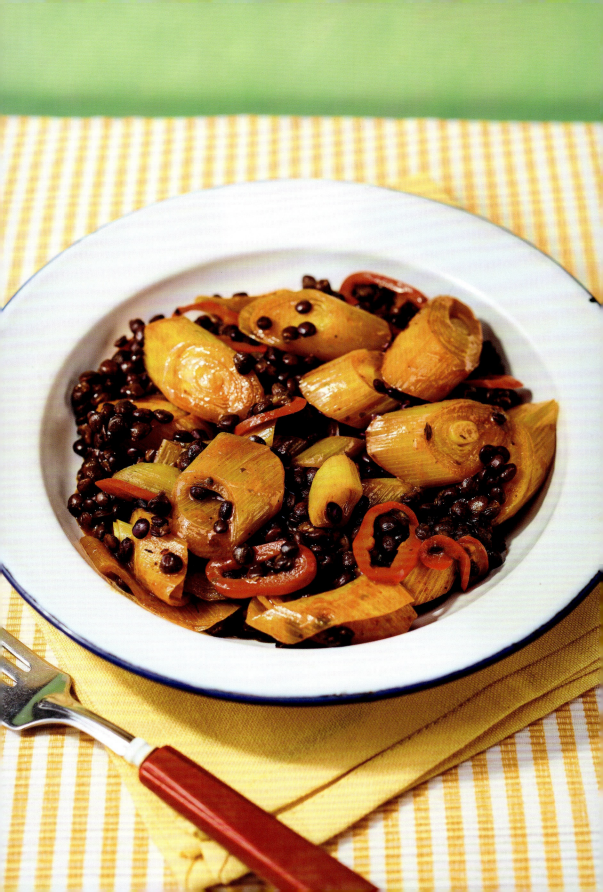

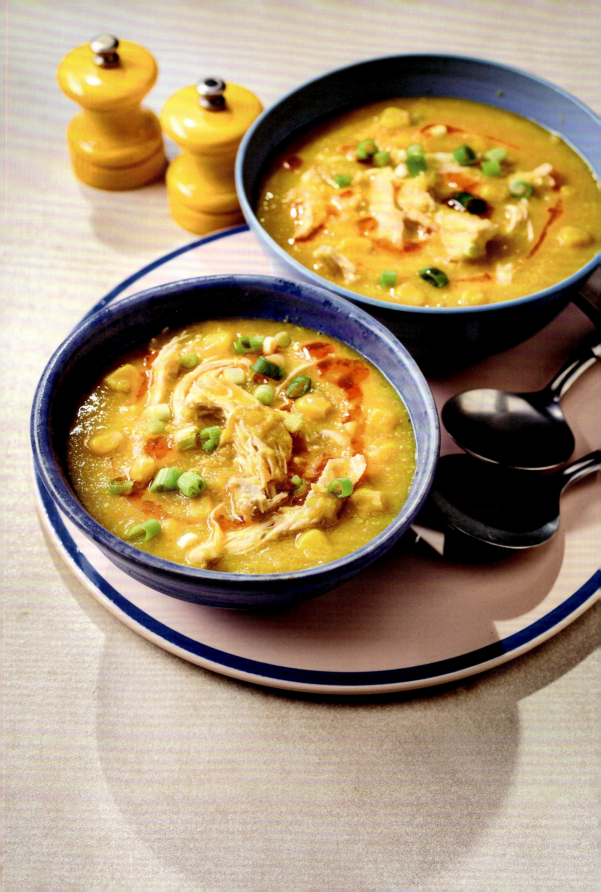

CHICKEN & SWEETCORN SOUP

262 CALORIES

SERVES 6

15 MINS

For me, this is a staple when ordering in a Chinese restaurant as it's simple and packs a ton of flavour. This is traditionally served with eggs (see Serving Note), so feel free to add these if you like.

4 x 400g tins of sweetcorn, drained

400g chicken breasts, whole

2 tbsp garlic and ginger paste

1 litre chicken stock

4 tbsp light soy sauce

1 tbsp sesame oil

1 Add three of the tins of sweetcorn to the slow cooker with all the remaining ingredients and some salt and pepper.

2 Cook on high for 3–4 hours or low for 6–7 hours, so it creates a gorgeous broth.

3 Remove the chicken to a plate and shred with two forks.

4 Blitz the broth and corn in the slow cooker with a hand blender, then stir in the shredded chicken and the remaining tin of sweetcorn.

5 Divide among bowls and garnish with a drizzle of oil (I love chilli oil) and some chopped spring onions, if you like.

SERVING NOTE:

I love cooking a plain egg omelette, then cutting it up into strips and adding it into the bowls for a different texture.

PROTEIN: 25g | **CARBS:** 26g | **FAT:** 6g

LOADED VEGETABLE SOUP

101 CALORIES

SERVES 8

15 MINS

A hugely nutritious soup that is perfect for the veg haters or for toddlers, as it's packed with goodness and loads of flavour. This is similar to a soup commonly served at Irish weddings.

3 leeks, roughly chopped

3 celery sticks, roughly chopped

4 carrots, peeled and roughly chopped

5 garlic cloves, roughly chopped

1 head of broccoli, roughly chopped

3 large potatoes, peeled and roughly chopped

1 Throw all the ingredients into the slow cooker with 1.2 litres of boiling water or vegetable stock and season with salt and pepper. Cook on high for 2–3 hours, then blitz in the slow cooker with a hand blender until smooth.

2 If you are feeling indulgent, stir through some cream and top with an extra sprinkle of pepper and some snipped fresh chives and/or some finely chopped red chilli for extra flavour and kick.

PROTEIN: 4g | **CARBS:** 17g | **FAT:** 1g

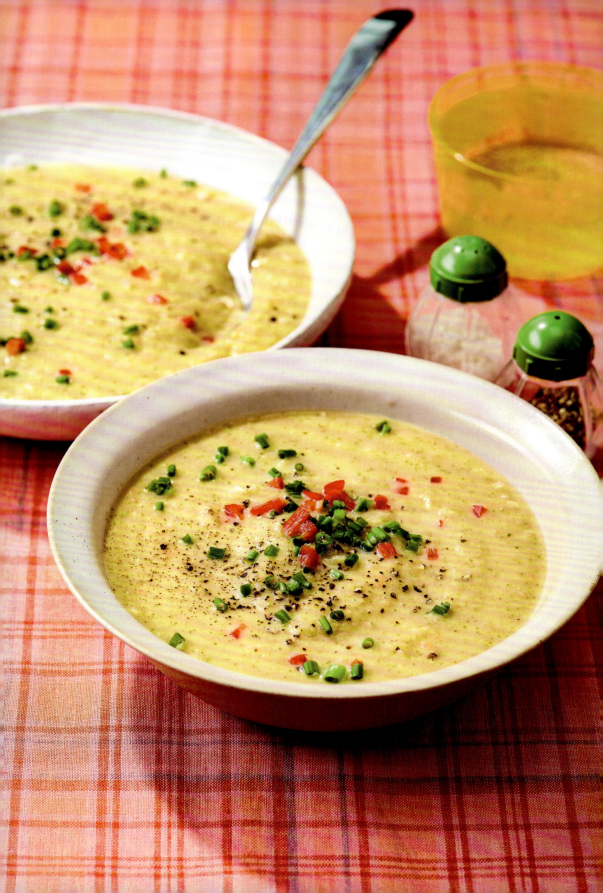

CURRIED CHORIZO, BACON & LENTIL SOUP

380 CALORIES

SERVES 6

10 MINS

This is incredibly moreish, with the bacon and chorizo fighting each other over who can be the dominant flavour in your mouth. Bring this soup to the office for lunch and everyone will be envious.

8 smoked streaky bacon rashers, chopped

200g chorizo, cubed

200g red split lentils, rinsed

700g passata

1½ tbsp curry paste of your choice

5 garlic cloves, grated

1 Briefly cook the bacon and chorizo in a hot pan until the bacon is golden – you can use a little oil if you aren't bothered about calories.

2 Add both meats to the slow cooker, along with all the other ingredients and 900ml of boiling water, then season with some salt and pepper. Cook on high for 2–3 hours or low for 5–6 hours. Check on the lentils an hour before the dish is ready and add more water if needed.

3 Ladle into bowls and grind over some more pepper.

SERVING NOTE:
Serve this with some chunks of crusty fresh bread.

PROTEIN: 23g | **CARBS:** 27g | **FAT:** 19g

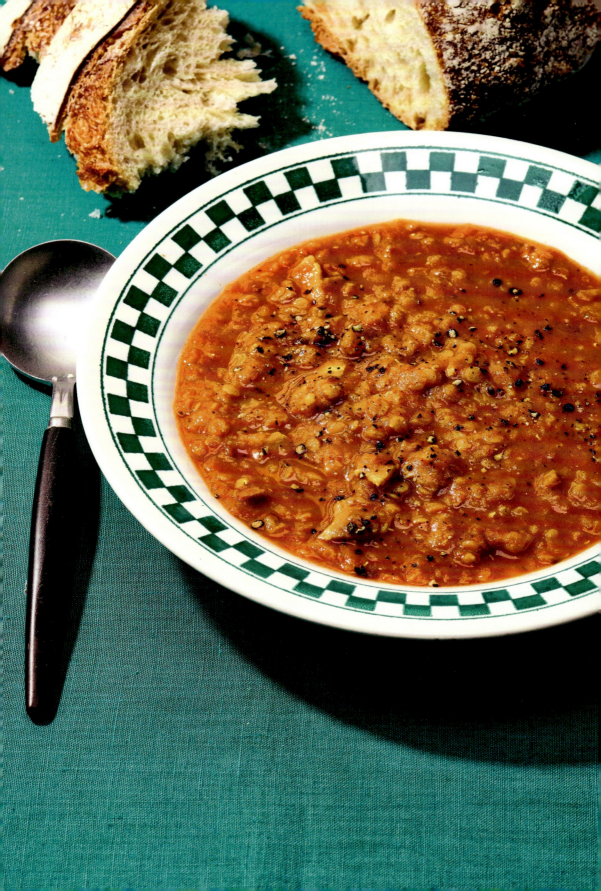

THROW & GO
SHARING DINNERS

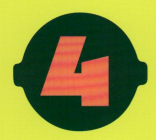

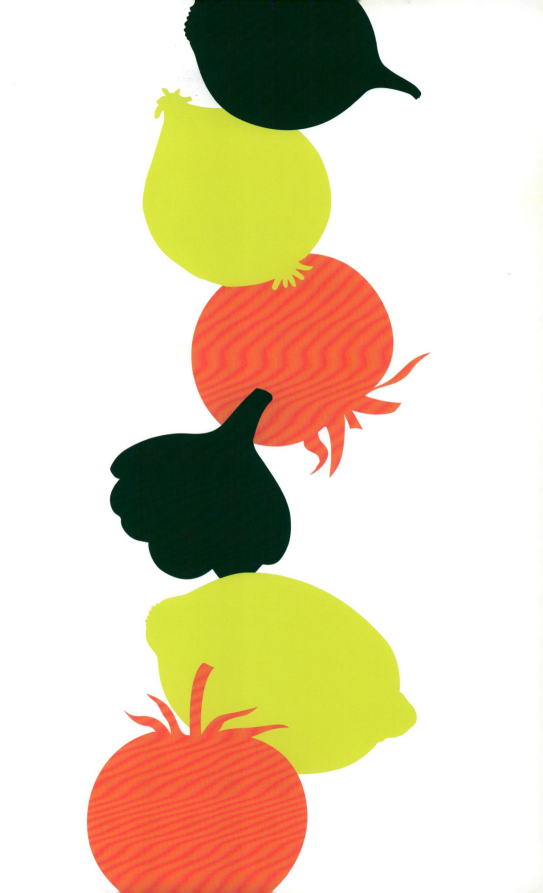

HARISSA LAMB SLIDERS

325 CALORIES

MAKES 12

15 MINS

I love making these when I'm feeding a crowd. I know I can throw everything in the slow cooker and come back to it later, without having to worry about prepping with everyone arriving. A real winner!

1.5kg boneless lamb shoulder

5 tbsp harissa paste

1 lemon, cut in half

12 mini slider buns, halved and toasted

300g reduced-fat coleslaw, to serve

4 pickles, sliced, to serve

1. Rub the lamb shoulder with the harissa and place it in the slow cooker. Add in the lemon halves and pour 200ml of boiling water or lamb stock all around. Cook on high for 4 hours or low for 8 hours until the lamb is completely tender.

2. Once cooked, remove the lamb to a plate and shred with two forks. Squeeze the lemon juices into the slow cooker and then remove and discard the lemon halves. Return the lamb to the slow cooker and stir through to coat in the juices.

3. Pile the warm shredded lamb onto the bottom halves of the toasted slider buns, then top with the coleslaw and pickles. Top with the bun lids and serve immediately.

PROTEIN: 29g | **CARBS:** 21g | **FAT:** 14g

Throw & Go Sharing Dinners

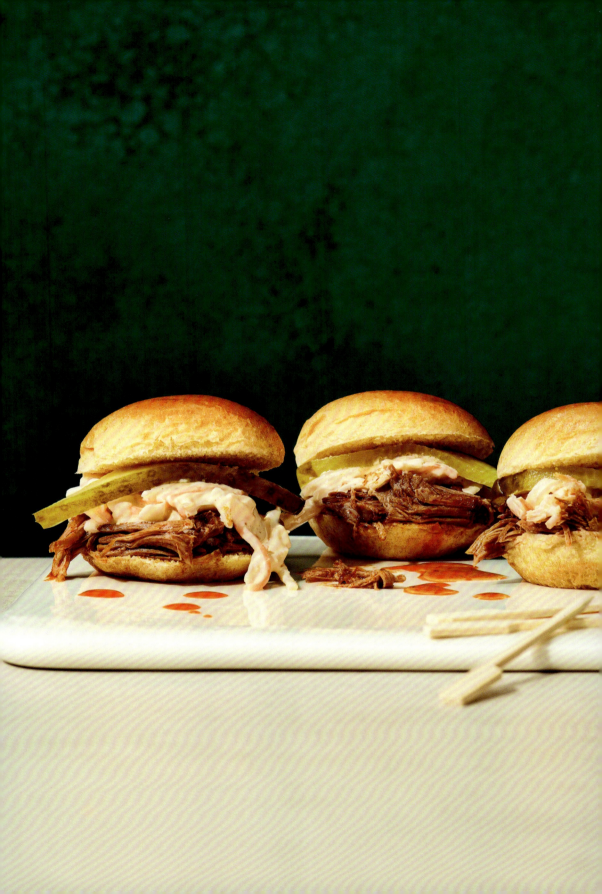

PULLED PORK & PINTO BEAN CHILLI WITH RICE

715 CALORIES

SERVES 6

10 MINS

I've always got a portion or two of this chilli in my freezer, as I get cravings for it. The smoky Cajun spices and slow-cooked peppers are the perfect match to the pulled pork and beans.

800g dried pinto beans, soaked overnight in cold water, then drained

800g boneless pork shoulder, cut into large chunks

2 tbsp smoky Cajun seasoning

500g passata

4 mixed red, orange and yellow peppers, thinly sliced

300g cooked white basmati rice, to serve

1 Place all the ingredients in the slow cooker, except the rice, and make sure the meat is completely covered with 500ml of boiling water or beef stock (add more if required). Cook on high for 4 hours or low for 8–10 hours until the beans are cooked through and the pork is completely tender.

2 Remove the pork to a plate and shred with two forks. Season the chilli with salt and pepper, then return the pulled pork to the chilli and serve with the rice.

SERVING NOTE:
To bulk this meal out, you could serve it with some tortilla chips, grated cheese, sliced avocado, sliced red chillies and lime wedges for squeezing over.

PROTEIN: 96g | **CARBS:** 61g | **FAT:** 9g

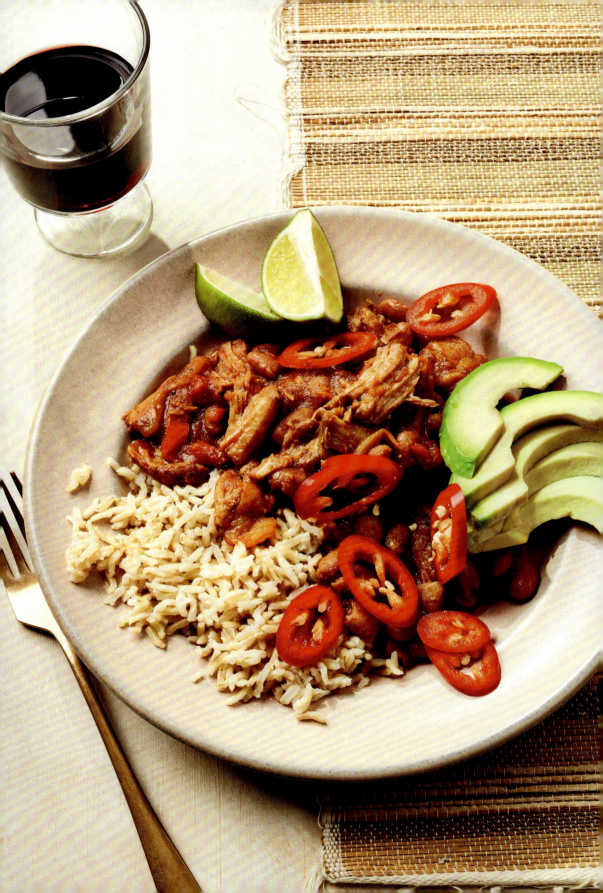

SOY & GINGER BRAISED SHORT RIBS

683 CALORIES

SERVES 4

15 MINS

If you really want to impress your guests, these ribs will do the trick. They will melt in the mouth and the sticky and rich sauce is just divine. I really have to stop myself from snacking on these before they reach my guests.

1.5kg beef short ribs
(around 4 ribs)

2 tbsp peeled and grated fresh ginger

100ml mirin

80ml light soy sauce

juice of 1 lemon or lime

100ml apple juice

1 Season the short ribs with salt and pepper and sear them on all sides in a large frying pan over a high heat with a little oil for a few minutes, then transfer to the slow cooker.

2 Add in all the remaining ingredients with 250ml of boiling water. Cook on high for 4 hours or low for 8 hours, or until the short ribs are completely tender. Turn the ribs around in the liquid a few times during cooking.

3 Once cooked, remove the short ribs to a serving platter and transfer the liquid to a saucepan. Bring to the boil and cook over a high heat until reduced to a glossy sauce consistency.

4 Drizzle the reduced sauce over the short ribs and serve with rice, some stir-fried pak choi, fresh coriander and sliced red chilli, if liked.

TIPS: *You can swap out the soy sauce and citrus juice for 100ml of ponzu if it's available.*

Short ribs can have a lot of fat, which will melt into your sauce. You can remove some of it by dropping a few ice cubes into the sauce before reducing, then skimming the fat off the top.

PROTEIN: 50g | **CARBS:** 24g | **FAT:** 43g

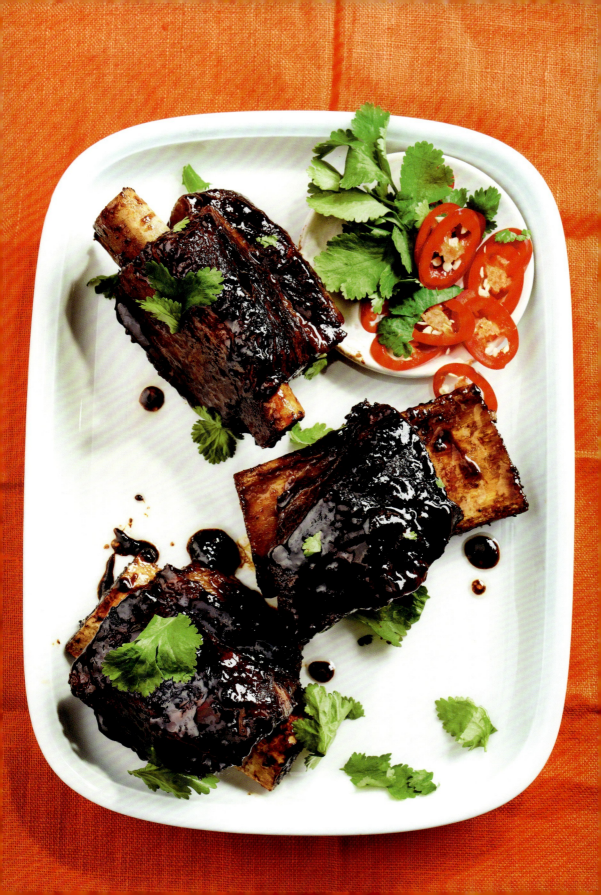

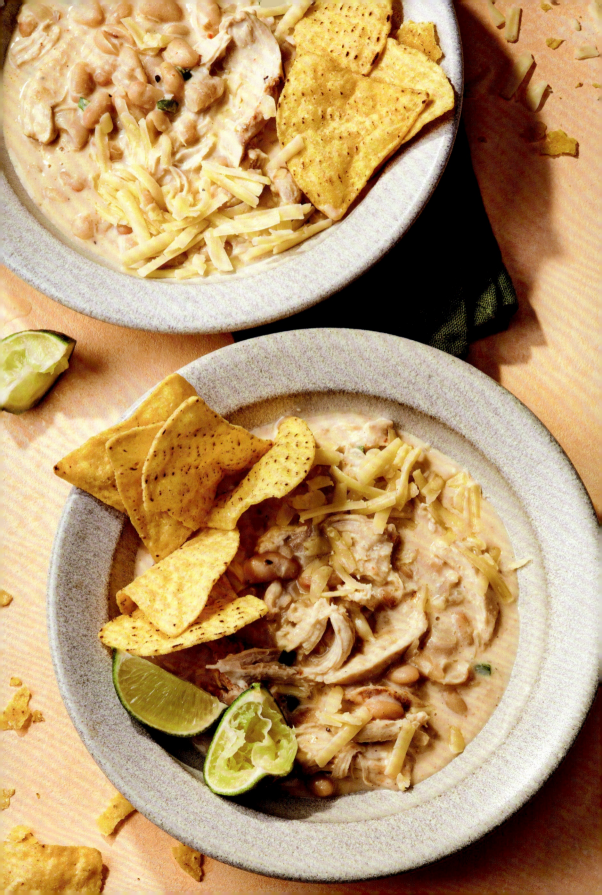

CHICKEN & BEAN WHITE CHILLI

279 CALORIES

SERVES 4

10 MINS

A chilli is so versatile, you can serve it with rice, tortilla chips or in a wrap. So many possibilities, but my favourite is when you've got all the extras to go with it – lime, Cheddar cheese, and even some soured cream.

1 onion, finely diced

2 fresh jalapeños, finely diced

2 tbsp Cajun seasoning

500g boneless and skinless chicken thighs or breasts, whole

400g tin of white beans, such as butter or cannellini, drained and rinsed

150g light soft cream cheese

1   Add all the ingredients, except the cream cheese, to the slow cooker. Add 250ml of boiling water or chicken stock, season with salt and pepper and cook on high for 3 hours or low for 6 hours.

2   Once the chicken is cooked, remove from the slow cooker to a plate and shred with two forks.

3   Season the sauce and stir through the cream cheese. Add the chicken back in and heat for 10–15 more minutes to warm through.

4   Serve immediately with your choice of sides.

SERVING NOTE:
Best served with some tortilla chips, grated Cheddar and lime wedges for squeezing over – yum!

PROTEIN: 37g | **CARBS:** 16g | **FAT:** 6g

LAMB WITH BALSAMIC VINEGAR

651 CALORIES

SERVES 4

15 MINS

I'd never eaten lamb with balsamic vinegar until I made this recipe, and now I'm never going back. The sweetness from the balsamic glaze works so well with the rich fattiness of the lamb.

1.5kg lamb shoulder, bone in

1 red onion, cut into wedges

4 garlic cloves, sliced

2 large sprigs of fresh rosemary, cut into smaller sprigs

500ml lamb or chicken stock

100ml balsamic vinegar (good-quality if possible)

1 Season and sear the lamb shoulder all over in a large frying pan over a high heat with a little oil.

2 Add the red onion wedges to the bottom of the slow cooker and place the seared lamb on top.

3 Cut deep holes all over the lamb and fill them with the sliced garlic, then scatter around the sprigs of rosemary. Add the stock and then drizzle over 50ml of the balsamic vinegar. Cook on high for 4 hours or low for 8 hours until the lamb is completely tender. When the lamb is cooked, remove it carefully from the slow cooker and allow to rest.

4 Heat the remaining balsamic vinegar in a small saucepan until reduced and treacle-like in texture. Add all the cooking juices from the slow cooker into another saucepan and heat until reduced to a gravy.

SERVING NOTE:
I love serving this with air-fried cubed potatoes and some green veg.

TIP: *Use leftover cold lamb to make wraps with pomegranate seeds and a cucumber yogurt.*

5 To serve, either leave the shoulder whole and drizzle over the reduction or remove the bone and shred the lamb using two forks. Drizzle over the balsamic reduction and serve with the gravy.

PROTEIN: 79g | **CARBS:** 10g | **FAT:** 32g

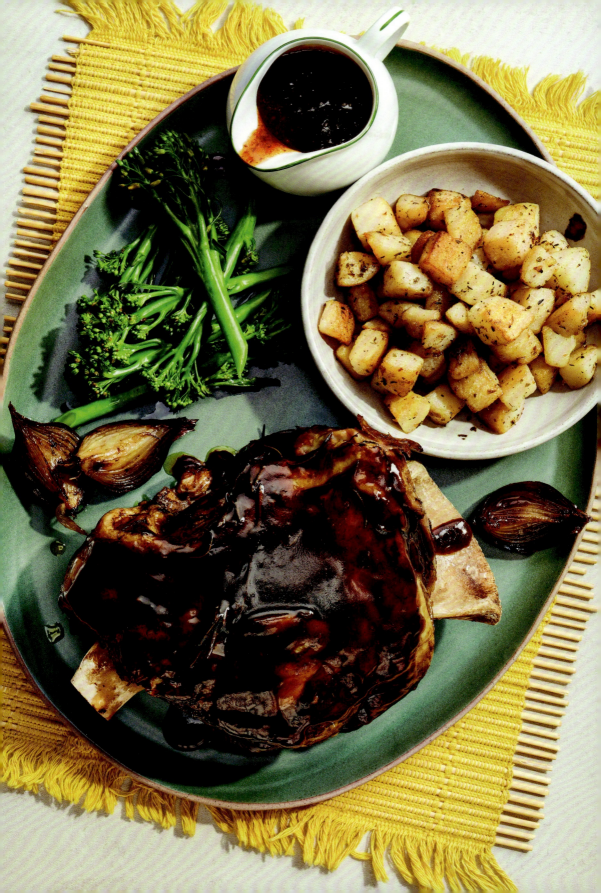

HONEY BBQ SHREDDED CHICKEN BURGERS

420 CALORIES

SERVES 4

10 MINS **(WITHOUT BUNS)**

These are great burgers – the perfect blend of sweet and tangy flavours – so gorgeous! But don't stop there, you could also use the filling for quick and tasty lunch wraps or even serve it with some rice for a super comforting meal that will have everyone asking for seconds.

4 chicken breasts, whole

100g BBQ sauce

50g honey

1 onion, finely diced

1 tbsp Worcestershire sauce

4 burger buns

1 Add all the ingredients, except the burger buns, to your slow cooker, season well with salt and pepper and add 150ml of boiling water or chicken stock. Cook on high for 4 hours or low for 8 hours until the chicken is cooked and tender.

2 Remove the chicken to a plate, then shred with two forks. Return to the slow cooker, season with salt and pepper and stir well to make sure the sauce covers everything.

3 Split and toast the burger buns and divide the chicken mixture between them.

PROTEIN: 42g | **CARBS:** 51g | **FAT:** 5g

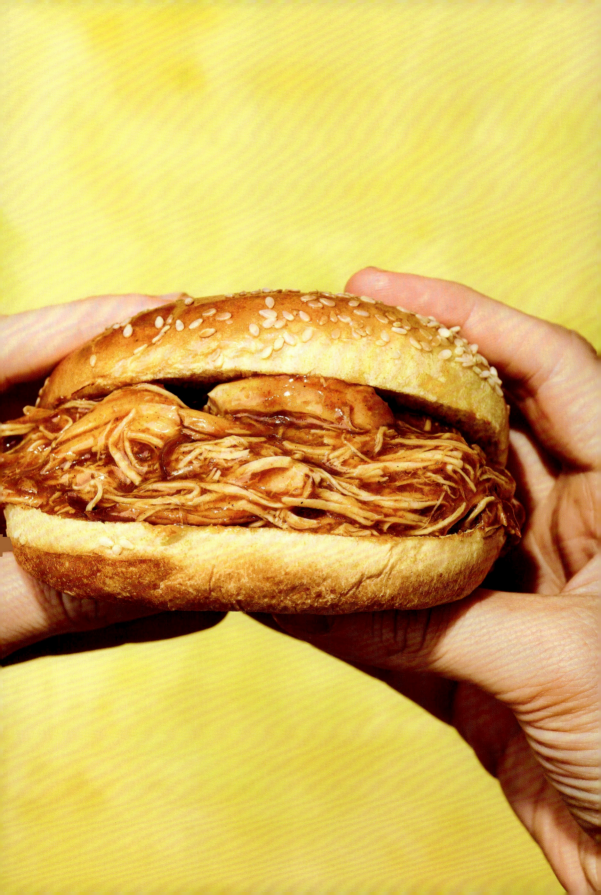

PESTO & PROSCIUTTO PORK WITH POTATOES

334 CALORIES

SERVES 6

10 MINS

Pork and mustard are a match made in heaven, but open that relationship to prosciutto and pesto and it becomes a whole other level of amazing. This is perfect if you're going out the door and want to feed the family quickly when you come home.

2 tbsp green pesto

2 tbsp Dijon mustard

700g pork tenderloin (in one piece)

120g prosciutto slices

700g baking potatoes, cubed, skin on

1 tbsp dried rosemary

1 In a bowl, combine the pesto and mustard, then cover the pork in this mixture. Wrap the pork tightly in the prosciutto slices so it is completely covered.

2 Add the cubed potatoes to the slow cooker with 100ml of boiling water or chicken stock and then place the pork tenderloin on top.

3 Drizzle the pork with 1 tablespoon of oil, then scatter over the dried rosemary and some salt and pepper. Cook on high for 4 hours or low for 7–8 hours until the pork is cooked and the potatoes are nicely browned and soft.

4 Slice the pork, then serve with the potatoes alongside. As well as the roast potato cubes, I love to serve this with peas – super simple and quick!

PROTEIN: 34g | **CARBS:** 27g | **FAT:** 12g

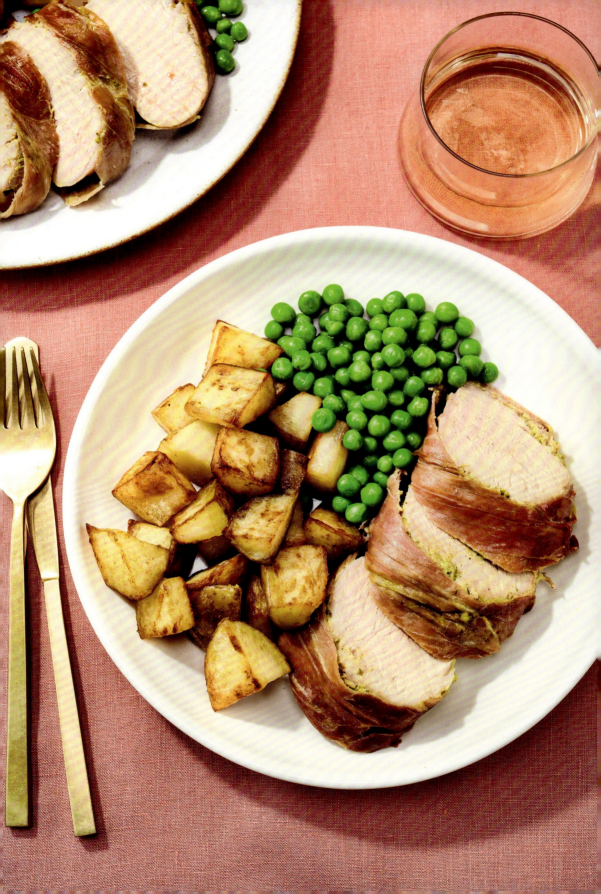

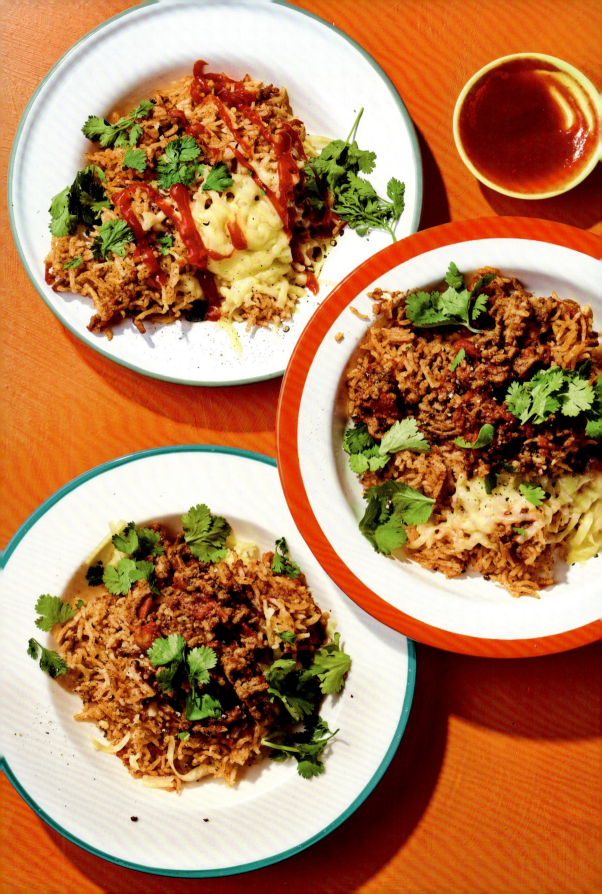

CHEESY BEEF TACO-STYLE RICE

495 CALORIES

SERVES 6

5 MINS

I love a taco in any form, but deconstructed and paired with rice and cheese, it is such a moreish meal and great for sharing. A total throw and go dish. While you can add more veg, garlic and herbs here, this really is all you need.

700g lean beef mince

25g sachet of taco seasoning

2 x 400g tins of chopped tomatoes

2 mixed peppers (red and yellow), thinly sliced

300g white basmati rice

100g reduced-fat Cheddar cheese, grated

1 Add all the ingredients to the slow cooker, apart from the rice and cheese, then cook on high for 3–4 hours or low for 7–8 hours.

2 Add the rice, 500ml of boiling water or beef stock and some salt and pepper, then cook for a further 45 minutes. Top with the cheese, close the lid and cook for a further 10–15 minutes.

3 You could serve this with some fresh coriander sprinkled on top, if liked. I also love to serve this with a good drizzle of chilli sauce.

PROTEIN: 36g | **CARBS:** 51g | **FAT:** 16g

WHOLE VINDALOO CHICKEN & POTATOES

417 CALORIES

SERVES 6

10 MINS

I will never get bored of lathering a whole chicken in a gorgeous curry paste and letting the meat draw in that flavour. Throw the potatoes under the chicken so they can cook in the chicken juices and that spiced curry heaven. A real showstopper!

800g baby potatoes, quartered

small handful of fresh coriander, chopped

3 garlic cloves, peeled but left whole

1 whole chicken (1.5kg minimum)

3 tbsp vindaloo curry paste (swap for a milder curry paste, if you like)

400ml tin of reduced-fat coconut milk

1 Add the potatoes to the bottom of the slow cooker with 100ml of boiling water or chicken stock, sprinkle with the coriander and throw in the whole garlic cloves.

2 Add in the chicken on top of the potatoes and coat it in the curry paste.

3 Cook on high for 4–5 hours or low for 7–8 hours.

4 For the last 30 minutes, gently stir in the coconut milk so it creates a curry/potato heaven situation and season with salt and pepper as needed.

5 Once it's ready, if you like, you can place the slow cooker pot (if it's ovenproof) under a hot grill for 7 minutes to crisp up the chicken skin before serving. Carve the chicken and serve with the potatoes and all the delicious juices.

PROTEIN: 48g | **CARBS:** 23g | **FAT:** 14g

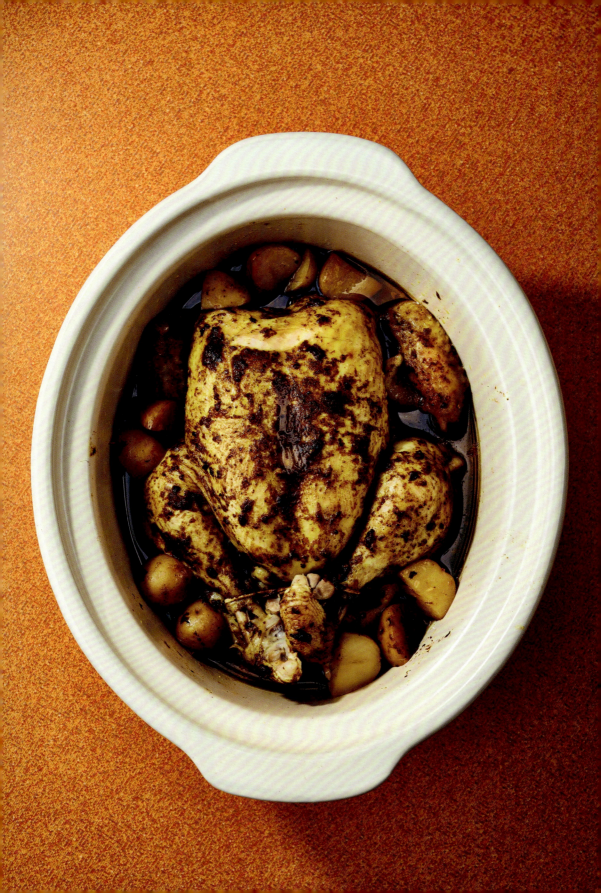

SUNDAY ROAST LAMB

387 CALORIES

SERVES 6

10 MINS

The easiest and most gorgeous lamb recipe with delicious juices to make that perfect gravy. This is ideal for Easter – while you eat your Easter eggs for breakfast, the slow cooker does all the hard work.

3 sprigs of fresh rosemary, cut into small pieces

small handful of fresh thyme leaves, finely chopped, plus extra to garnish

1 tsp paprika

1 tsp onion granules

3 garlic cloves, peeled but left whole

1.2kg leg of lamb

1 Put the fresh herbs in a bowl and add the paprika, onion granules, some salt and pepper and 2 tablespoons of oil. Mix this together into a paste and use it to coat the lamb generously.

2 Add the garlic and lamb to the slow cooker with 100ml of boiling water or lamb stock and cook on high for 6–7 hours or low for 10–12 hours until the lamb is very tender.

3 Pour the juices into a saucepan (keeping the garlic cloves with the lamb) and cook until reduced to a gravy. Serve the lamb and garlic with the gravy, and scatter over a few extra thyme leaves to finish.

PROTEIN: 42g | **CARBS:** 0g | **FAT:** 24g

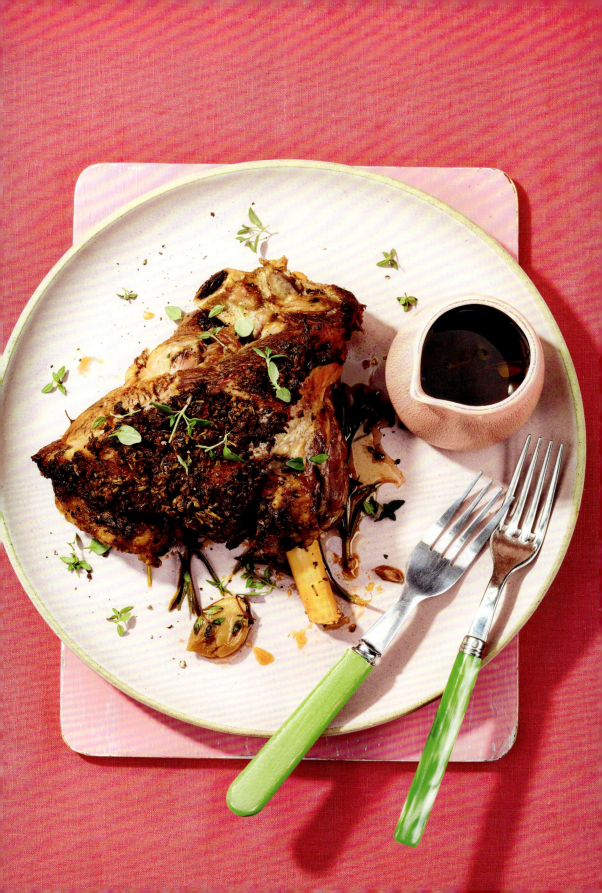

IRISH SAVOURY MINCE & CARROTS

240 CALORIES

SERVES 6

10 MINS

This is a childhood classic for me, as my granda always made this and the only way to have it is with mash and peas. It feels a bit like a deconstructed cottage pie, and I love it. All the nostalgia with none of the hard work.

600g lean beef mince

4 carrots, peeled and cut into small cubes or chunks

1 rich beef stock pot

4 tbsp Worcestershire sauce

4 tbsp tomato purée

4 garlic cloves, crushed

1 You can brown the mince in a frying pan with 1 tablepoon of oil over a high heat, but it's not essential. If you don't brown it, cut it up with scissors so it doesn't clump. Add the mince and all the other ingredients to the slow cooker, season with salt and pepper and add 450ml of boiling water. Cook on high for 3–4 hours or low for 7–8 hours.

2 If you want a thick sauce, add 2 tablespoons of cornflour mixed with 2 tablespoons of water, or some gravy granules. I prefer gravy granules or powder. Cook the mince on high for a further 20–30 minutes.

3 Serve the savoury mince with some side dishes.

SERVING NOTE:
Mashed potatoes, peas (my fave) or broccoli are a must.

PROTEIN: 23g | **CARBS:** 9g | **FAT:** 12g

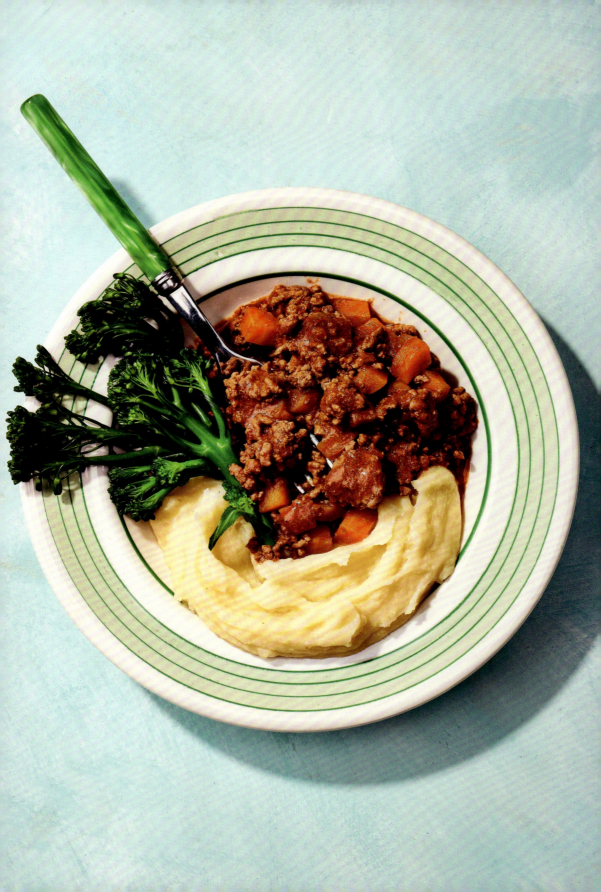

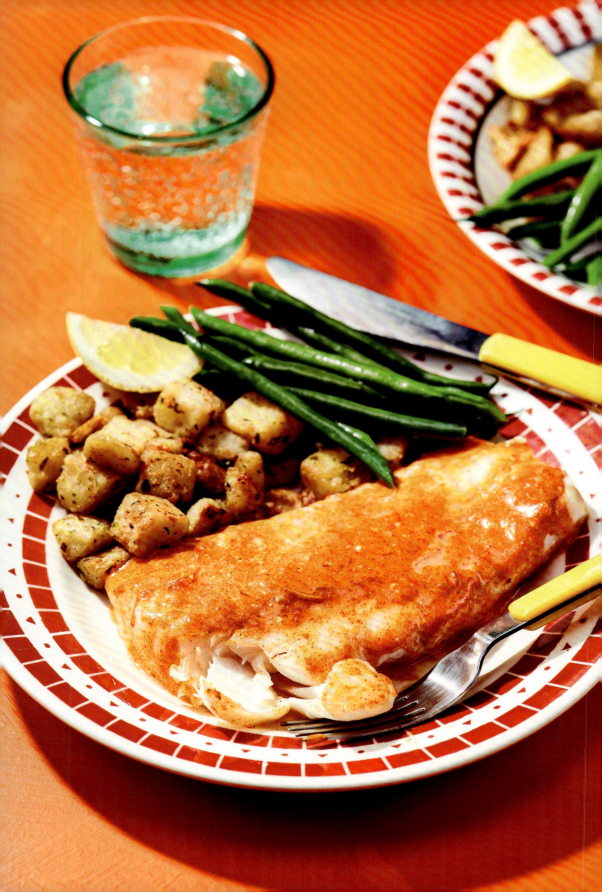

LEMON PAPRIKA COD

150 CALORIES

SERVES 4

5 MINS

Fish cooked in the slow cooker is perfection, as it spends the hours soaking up the flavour and leaves you with a flaky rich fish that works really well with any side.

4 cod fillets (I prefer skinless)

1½ tbsp paprika

2 lemons, 1 juiced and 1 cut into slices

2 garlic cloves, grated

200ml fish or chicken stock

1 tbsp half-fat crème fraîche

1　Coat the cod in the paprika, then add to the slow cooker with all the other ingredients, except the crème fraîche. Add 1 tablespoon of butter or oil and cook on high for 1–2 hours or low for 3–4 hours.

2　After this time, gently remove the cod to a plate, then stir the crème fraîche into the sauce and season with salt and pepper. Add 1 tablespoon of cornflour mixed with 1 tablespoon of water to thicken and cook on high for another 20 minutes, if required.

3　Pour the sauce over the fish and serve with your sides of choice.

SERVING NOTE:
I like to serve this with air-fried cubed potatoes, green beans and some lemon wedges for squeezing over.

PROTEIN: 26g　|　**CARBS:** 0g　|　**FAT:** 5g

CREAMY BEEF & MUSHROOM ORZOTTO

465 CALORIES

SERVES 4

5 MINS

If you close your eyes this would trick you into thinking a stroganoff and risotto jumped into a pot together. I could eat orzo every day, and from what I hear from my online followers, a lot of you love it for weaning recipes, too.

350g beef rump or thin steaks, cut into strips

300g chestnut mushrooms, cut in half

3 garlic cloves, grated

3 tbsp Worcestershire sauce

270g dried orzo

2 tbsp half-fat crème fraîche

1 Add all the ingredients to the slow cooker, except the orzo and crème fraîche, and add in 40g of butter or oil and 100ml of boiling water. Cook on high for 3–4 hours or low for 6 hours.

2 After this time, stir in the orzo and 650ml of boiling water and season with salt and pepper, then close the lid and cook on high for a further 1 hour. Stir in the crème fraîche, then serve with an extra grind or two of pepper.

PROTEIN: 28g | **CARBS:** 55g | **FAT:** 14g

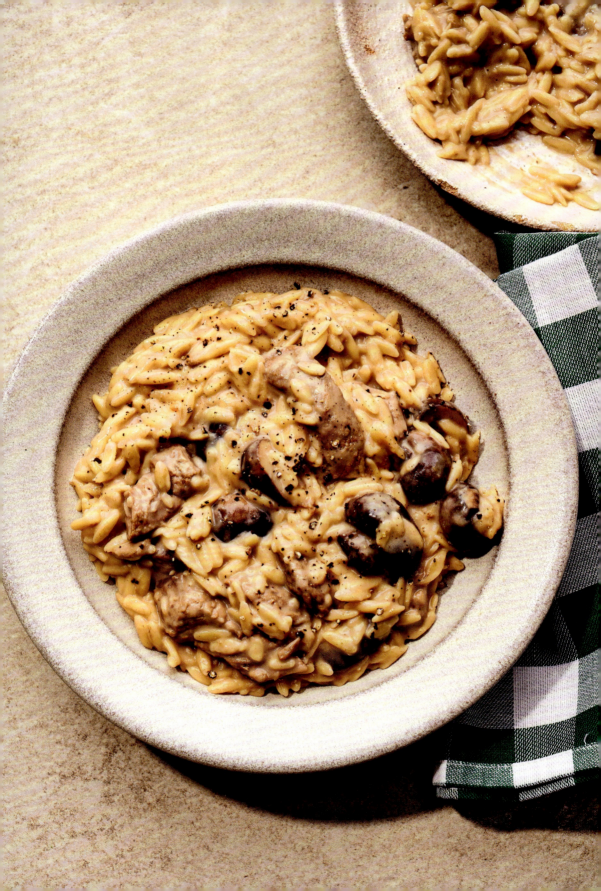

SWEET POTATO & LENTIL SHEPHERD'S PIE

489 CALORIES

SERVES 6

20 MINS

Incredibly filling and full of goodness, with sweet potato in both the filling and the mash topping. The addition of red pesto and fresh thyme allows you to pack in so much flavour with so few ingredients.

2kg sweet potatoes, peeled and chopped into cubes

3 x 400g tins of chopped tomatoes

2 x 400g tins of lentils, drained and rinsed

4 tbsp vegetarian garlicky red pesto

bunch of fresh thyme, leaves picked and finely chopped, plus extra for the mash

2 tsp dried rosemary

1   Add 1kg of the sweet potatoes to the slow cooker along with all the other ingredients. Add some salt and pepper and 100ml of boiling water. Cook on high for 2–3 hours or low for 4–5 hours.

2   Before this is ready, make some mash by cooking the remaining sweet potatoes in a pan of boiling water until soft. Drain and mash with a couple of good knobs of butter and some extra chopped thyme, then spread this over the top of the pie filling. You could sprinkle some finely grated Cheddar cheese on top, if you like.

3   Pop under a hot grill for 10–12 minutes until the topping is nice and crisp. If your slow cooker pot isn't ovenproof, transfer to another dish before grilling.

TIP: *This is a veggie pie, but you could swap in 500g of beef (or lamb) mince instead of the sweet potatoes and just have the sweet potato mash topping.*

PROTEIN: 14g | **CARBS:** 93g | **FAT:** 5g

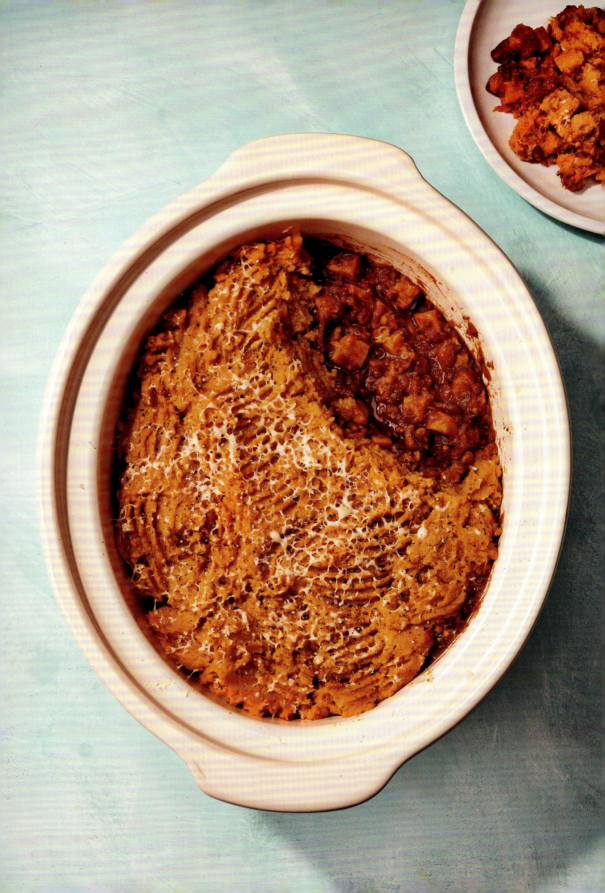

BRAISED DAUBE OF BEEF IN A PORT GRAVY

381 CALORIES

SERVES 6

10 MINS

This delicious crowd-pleasing beef dish is sure to win everyone over. It's no secret that port, wine – or both – added to a gravy makes it incredibly rich and delicious.

1.2kg beef chuck, cut into large cubes

25ml port

1 rich beef stock pot

300ml red wine

small handful of fresh rosemary, leaves picked and chopped, plus extra leaves to garnish

4 garlic cloves, crushed

1 Season the beef with salt and pepper and sear all over in a hot pan with 1 tablespoon of oil for a few minutes.

2 Add to the slow cooker with all the other ingredients and 100ml of boiling water. Cook on high for 4–5 hours or low for 7–8 hours.

3 Add 1–2 tablespoons of cornflour mixed with 1 tablespoon of water to the sauce and cook on high for 20–30 minutes until thickened.

4 Serve the braised beef with the gravy on top and sprinkled with a few extra rosemary leaves to finish.

SERVING NOTE:
Serve the braised beef on top of a lovely buttery mash or colcannon with some seasonal green veg alongside.

PROTEIN: 44g | **CARBS:** 6g | **FAT:** 13g

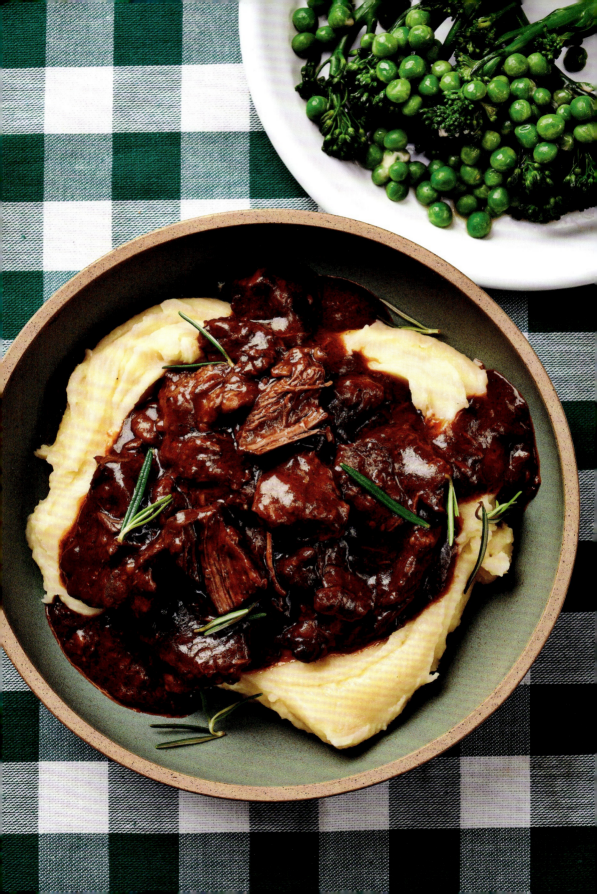

SET & FORGET
MIDWEEK MEALS

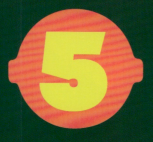

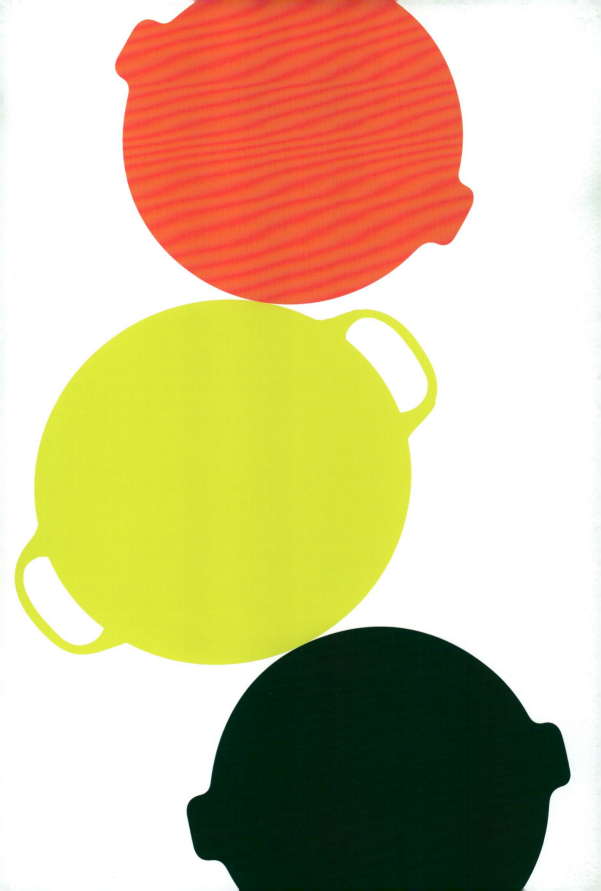

MARRY ME CHICKEN MADE EASY

432 CALORIES

SERVES 4

10 MINS

This is one of those viral trends, and apparently if you make it for someone, they will want to marry you. While it does taste amazing, and I have made it many times, I am not married yet (at the time of writing), so I'm not sure it fully works, but you will love it. This is a stripped-back version using fewer ingredients, so you can make it with very little in the house.

2 tbsp Cajun seasoning, or paprika

4 chicken breasts, whole

4 handfuls of sundried tomatoes, roughly chopped

generous handful of fresh basil leaves, plus extra to garnish

2 tbsp dried mixed Italian herbs

100ml double cream

1 Mix 2 tablespoons of cornflour with 1 tablespoon of the Cajun seasoning, and season with salt and pepper. Coat the chicken breasts in this mix.

2 Add 2 tablespoons of oil to a frying pan and, once hot, seal the chicken for 1–2 minutes on each side.

3 Add the chicken to the slow cooker. Add all the other ingredients, apart from the cream, along with 300ml of boiling water or chicken stock. Cook on high for 3–4 hours or low for 7–8 hours.

4 Stir in the cream and serve with your sides of choice and garnish with an extra grind of pepper and a few more basil leaves.

SERVING NOTE:

This goes well with orzo pasta or rice.

PROTEIN: 37g | **CARBS:** 10g | **FAT:** 30g

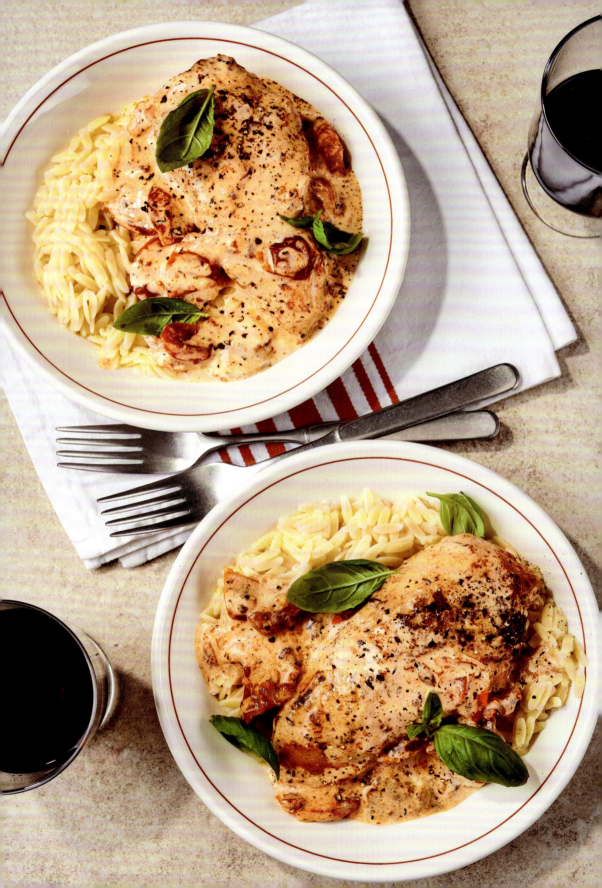

CREAMY CHICKEN MEATBALLS WITH GNOCCHI

502 CALORIES

SERVES 4

10 MINS

Gnocchi and meatballs are two of my favourite ingredients, so why not throw them together to make this delicious dish? It's super rich and creamy, and great for a midweek dinner.

500g lean chicken thigh mince

50g fresh white breadcrumbs

250g passata

50ml double cream

500g ready-made fresh gnocchi

50g Parmesan cheese, finely grated, plus extra to serve

1 Combine the chicken mince and breadcrumbs with some salt and pepper and then form into 16–20 meatballs. Place in the slow cooker with the passata and 150ml of boiling water or chicken stock. Season well and cook on high for 3 hours.

2 Once the meatballs are cooked through, remove to a baking tray. Add the double cream, gnocchi and grated Parmesan to the slow cooker, then cook on high for 30 minutes.

3 Meanwhile, place the meatballs under a hot grill and cook for 4–5 minutes, or until they have a little char and are golden-coloured. Keep warm.

4 Once the gnocchi are cooked, return the meatballs to the slow cooker, stir well to combine, then serve immediately, sprinkled with a grind of pepper and some extra Parmesan. Garnish with a few fresh basil leaves, too.

PROTEIN: 39g | **CARBS:** 50g | **FAT:** 15g

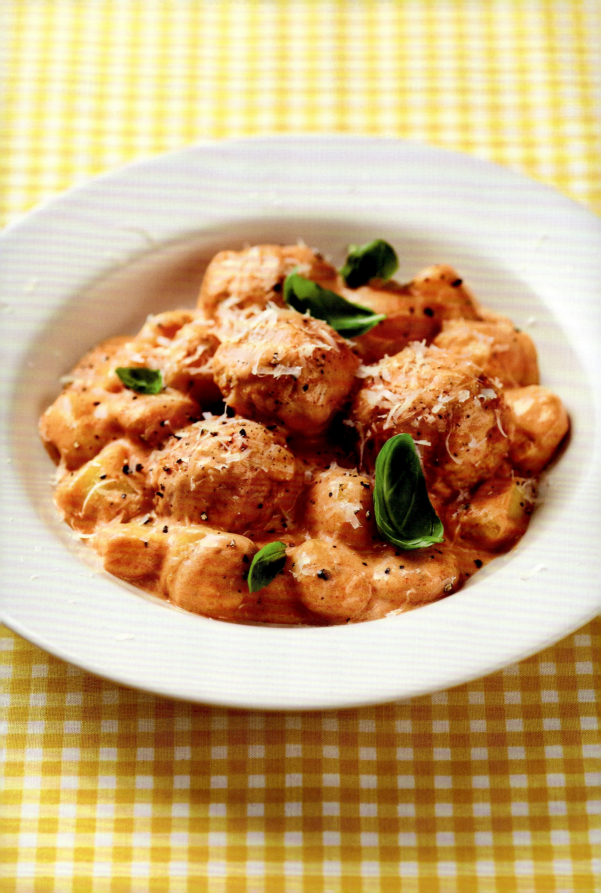

DUCK PILAF

679 CALORIES

SERVES 4

10 MINS

Duck legs are beautiful in the slow cooker, because the slow-cooked meat falls off the bone and melts in your mouth. If you don't have duck legs, you can always use large chicken legs.

4 duck legs, skin on

250g white basmati rice

1 onion, thinly sliced

1 tbsp coriander seeds, whole

1 cinnamon stick

handful of fresh mint leaves, shredded

1   Place the duck legs in the slow cooker with 500ml of boiling water or chicken stock and cook on high for 4 hours or low for 8 hours until completely tender. Remove from the stock, discard the skin and shred the meat from the bones using two forks, then set aside.

2   Tip the basmati rice into a sieve and rinse well until the water runs clear, then add to the stock in the slow cooker with the onion, coriander seeds, some salt and pepper and the cinnamon stick. Close the lid and cook on high for 1 hour, or until the rice has absorbed all the liquid and is cooked through and tender.

3   Reheat the shredded duck for 1 minute in the microwave and then add it back to the slow cooker, remove the cinnamon stick and stir well. You can grill the pilaf briefly now (if the slow cooker pot is ovenproof) if you want to crisp up the top, but it's not essential.

4   Top with the shredded mint leaves and serve.

SERVING NOTE:
You could even scatter over some pomegranate seeds for extra flavour and colour.

PROTEIN: 61g | **CARBS:** 53g | **FAT:** 24g

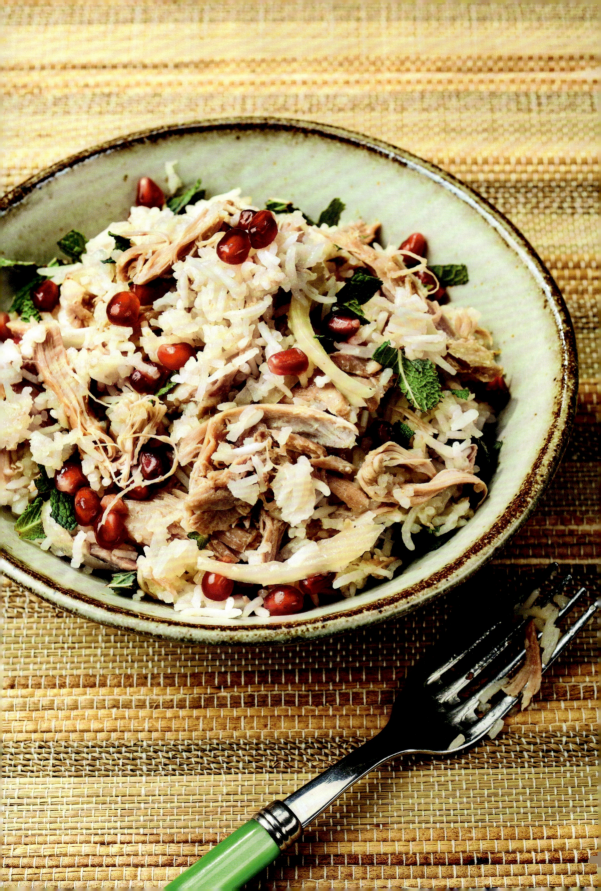

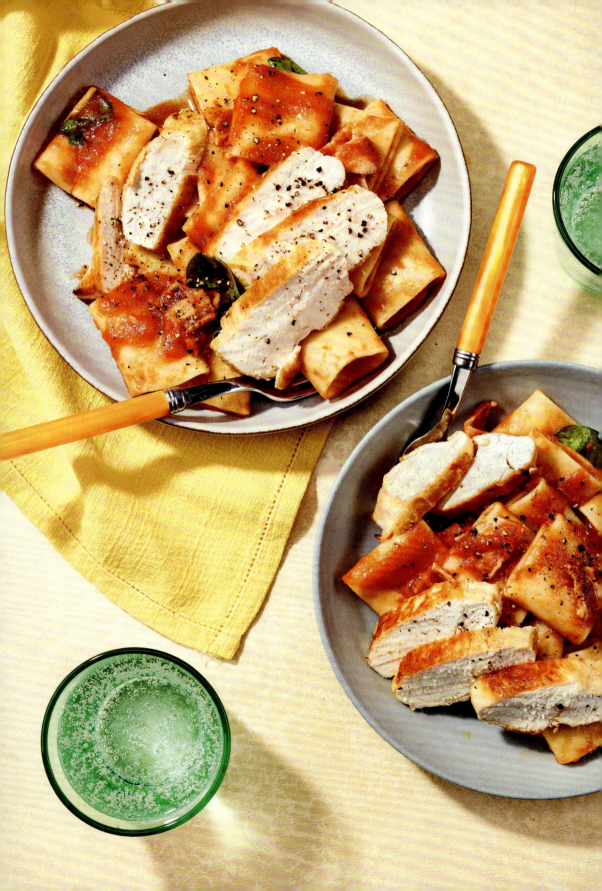

TOMATO, BACON & BASIL CHICKEN PASTA

574 CALORIES

SERVES 4

10 MINS

Throw your chicken into this tomato, bacon and herb bath and let it do its thing all day. You don't have to serve with pasta, potatoes and veg would also work brilliantly. That's the versatility of these recipes, customise them to suit your taste.

8 smoked streaky bacon rashers, chopped

4 chicken breasts, whole

800g passata

handful of fresh basil leaves, plus extra to garnish

4 garlic cloves, sliced

500g cooked pasta of your choice

1   Brown the bacon and chicken all over in a hot frying pan for a few minutes in 1 tablespoon of oil, then add to the slow cooker with all the other ingredients, except the pasta, adding some salt and pepper. Cook on high for 4 hours or low for 8 hours.

2   Once cooked, stir through the pasta and slice the chicken if preferred. Top with more fresh basil and enjoy.

PROTEIN: 53g | **CARBS:** 55g | **FAT:** 14g

CHICKPEA, POTATO & CHORIZO STEW

538 CALORIES

SERVES 4

10 MINS

Anything with chorizo in it and I will have it. If you aren't a chorizo lover, just use flavourful pork sausages and remove the skin, then break up into small pieces. This stew really packs a flavour punch with so few ingredients.

300g chorizo, sliced

600g baby potatoes, cut in half

400g tin of chickpeas, drained and rinsed

4 garlic cloves, crushed

2 tbsp curry paste of your choice

3 handfuls of baby spinach leaves

1 Pan-fry the chorizo in 1 tablespoon of oil over a high heat for a few minutes. Add about three-quarters of the chorizo to the slow cooker (reserve the rest to serve – see Tip) with all the other ingredients, apart from the spinach. Add 400ml of boiling water or chicken stock, then cook on high for 4 hours or low for 7 hours.

2 For the last 5 minutes of the cooking time, stir through the spinach to wilt and season with more salt and pepper, if needed. Serve the stew in bowls topped with some of the reserved (finely chopped) crispy chorizo, so you have a lovely crunch when you tuck in.

TIP: *I chop the reserved crispy chorizo for serving into small chunks like little lardons. Make sure you leave it to cool and then refrigerate it before reheating it when you serve.*

PROTEIN: 26g | **CARBS:** 37g | **FAT:** 31g

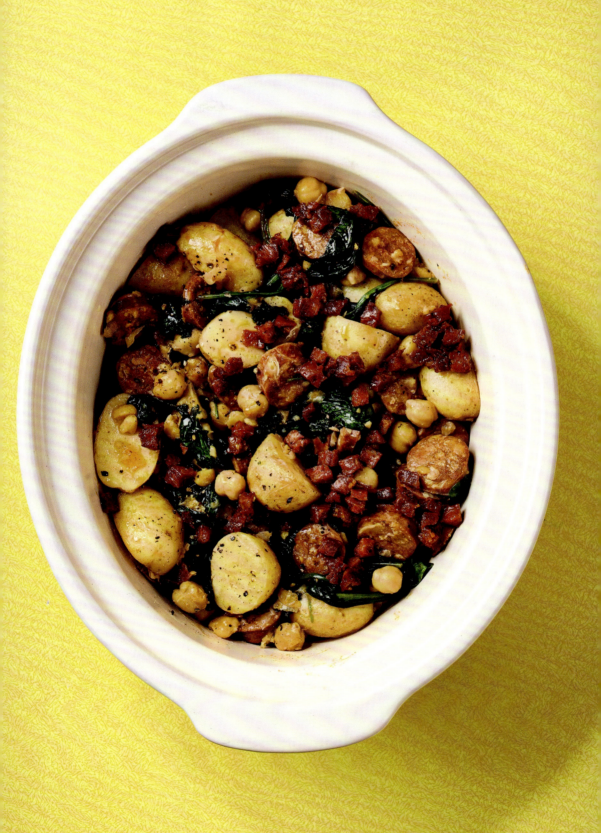

GOCHUJANG HONEY RIBS

623 CALORIES

SERVES 4

15 MINS

These ribs fall off the bone and the sauce is the perfect balance of sweet and spicy that will keep you coming back for more. I honestly could devour these in minutes.

1.5kg meaty pork ribs

4 tbsp gochujang paste
(alternatively use sriracha or another chilli paste/sauce)

4 tbsp honey

50ml light soy sauce

1 tbsp garlic and ginger paste

1 tbsp sesame seeds

1   Place all the ingredients, except the sesame seeds, into the slow cooker with around 750ml of boiling water or chicken stock to cover the ribs. Cook on high for 4 hours or low for 8 hours until the meat is completely tender.

2   Remove the ribs, place them on a baking tray and cut them up into individual ribs. Transfer the juices to a saucepan and boil until reduced, thick and glossy. Drizzle the sauce over the ribs, then pop under a hot grill until they crisp up. Serve hot with sesame seeds sprinkled on top. You could also add some sliced spring onion, if you like.

PROTEIN: 52g | **CARBS:** 26g | **FAT:** 34g

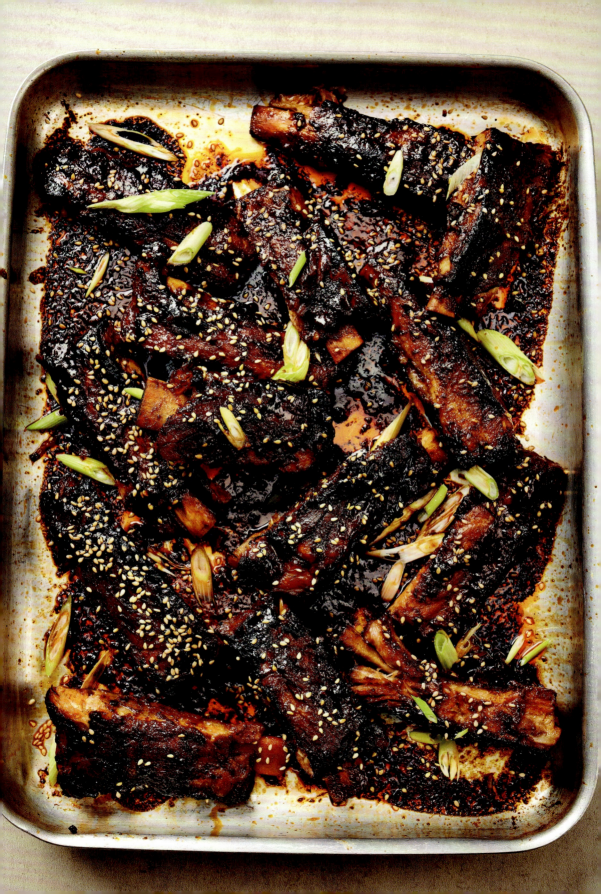

CREAMY BUTTERNUT SQUASH & LEMON LINGUINE

544 CALORIES

SERVES 4

10 MINS

This gorgeous veggie linguine, with the flavour of lemon punching through, plus a good glug of cream, is all you need for those weekdays when you fancy a tasty meatless meal.

1kg frozen butternut squash cubes

4 garlic cloves, grated

zest and juice of 1 large lemon or 2 small lemons

handful of fresh sage leaves, chopped, plus extra leaves to garnish

350g dried linguine

100ml double cream

1 Put all the ingredients into the slow cooker, apart from the pasta and cream, and add 100ml of boiling water or vegetable stock and some salt and pepper. Cook on high for 2–3 hours or low for 4–5 hours.

2 Towards the end of the cooking time, cook the linguine in a pan of boiling water until al dente, then drain and reserve some of the cooking water.

3 Blitz the sauce in the slow cooker with a hand blender, and if it needs loosening, add a few tablespoons of the reserved pasta water.

4 Stir through the warm cooked linguine and cream, close the lid and heat for 2–3 minutes on high, then serve garnished with an extra grind of pepper and the sage leaves.

PROTEIN: 13g | **CARBS:** 87g | **FAT:** 15g

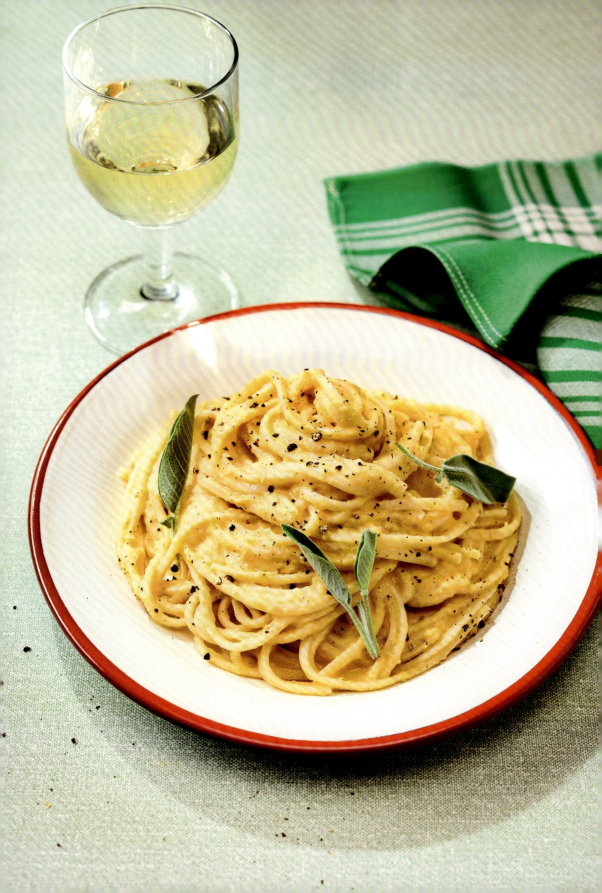

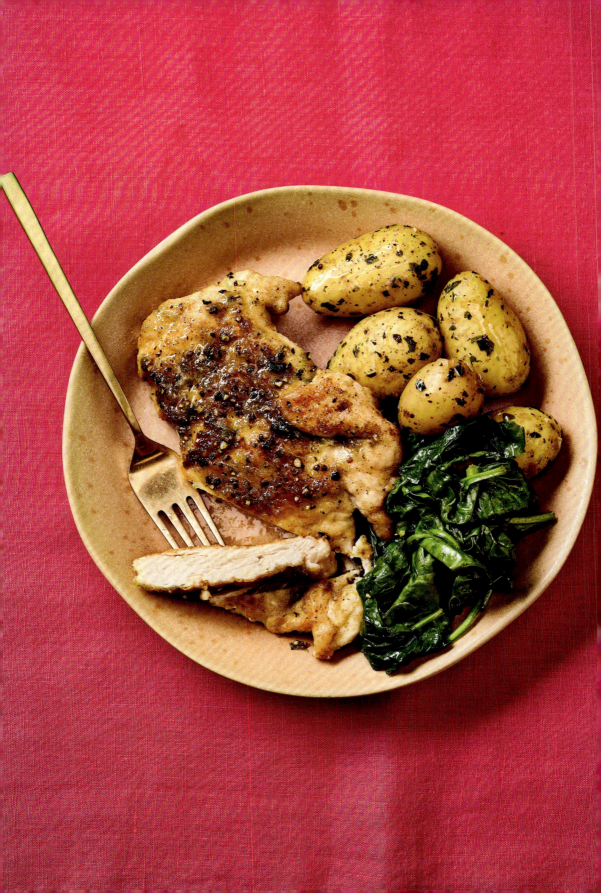

LEMON, BLACK PEPPER & BUTTER CHICKEN

377 CALORIES

SERVES 4

10 MINS

This simple classic goes perfectly with whatever you choose to pair it with, whether that be baby new potatoes or pasta. It's divine and perfect for a midweek meal.

4 chicken breasts, whole

120g half-fat butter

juice of 1 lemon, plus 2 slices of lemon

1 tsp black peppercorns, crushed

4 garlic cloves, crushed

1 tbsp honey

1. Flatten the chicken breasts with a rolling pin, then coat in around 1 tablespoon of flour or cornflour. Sear in a hot frying pan in 1 tablespoon of oil for 1 minute on each side.

2. Add the seared chicken to the slow cooker with all the remaining ingredients, 50ml of boiling water or chicken stock and some salt and pepper. Cook on high for 3–4 hours or low for 6–7 hours.

3. Serve the buttery lemon-pepper chicken breasts with your favourite sides.

SERVING NOTE:
Herby new potatoes with some wilted spinach or greens will work a treat.

PROTEIN: 36g | **CARBS:** 7g | **FAT:** 18g

FETA, TOMATO & RED PEPPER PASTA

339 CALORIES

SERVES 4

10 MINS

You remember it, don't you? That viral trend where feta was out of stock everywhere because this pasta dish was having its moment. This is my version with a twist, made in the slow cooker with roasted red peppers and cherry tomatoes.

20 cherry tomatoes

1 x 375g jar of roasted red peppers, drained

4 garlic cloves, crushed or grated

1 x 200g block of reduced-fat feta cheese

handful of fresh basil leaves, plus extra to garnish

500g cooked pasta (I like fusilli)

1 Add the tomatoes, red peppers and garlic to the slow cooker, set the whole block of feta in among the veg and add 1–2 tablespoons of water with the basil leaves, then season well with salt and pepper. Cook on high for 2½ hours or low for 4 hours.

2 Blitz to a sauce in the slow cooker with a hand blender, then stir in the cooked pasta and serve, garnished with an extra grind or two of pepper and some more basil leaves.

PROTEIN: 17g | **CARBS:** 51g | **FAT:** 7g

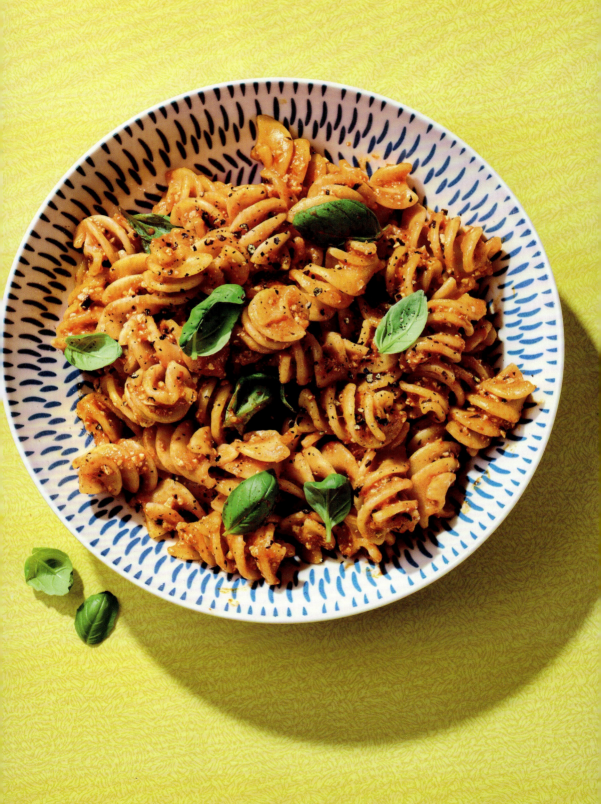

MEATBALL SUB BAKE WITH CRISPY CROUTONS

572 CALORIES

SERVES 4

10 MINS

We've done the meatball sub, now we have the sub bake – even easier and perfect for a midweek meal! The croutons give this dish a great crunch that contrasts with the soft meatballs and gooey yet crispy cheese.

400g ready-made lean beef or pork meatballs

500g passata

1 onion, finely chopped

3 garlic cloves, crushed

4 sub rolls

100g reduced-fat Cheddar cheese, grated

1 Add the meatballs, passata, onion and garlic to the slow cooker, along with 100ml of boiling water or beef stock, and cook on high for 3 hours or low for 6 hours.

2 An hour before the meatballs are cooked, tear up the sub rolls into bited-size pieces, place on a baking tray and toss with a tablespoon of oil and some salt and pepper. Toast in a preheated oven or air fryer at 200°C for about 10 minutes until crisp and golden. Add the croutons on top of the meatball mix to soak up some of the sauce, then top with the grated cheese and cook on high for 30 minutes.

3 Once the meatballs are cooked, place the slow cooker dish (as long as it's ovenproof – if not, decant the mixture into a baking dish) under a hot grill to crisp up the croutons and Cheddar. Serve immediately. You could even garnish with some fresh basil leaves too.

PROTEIN: 33g | **CARBS:** 42g | **FAT:** 30g

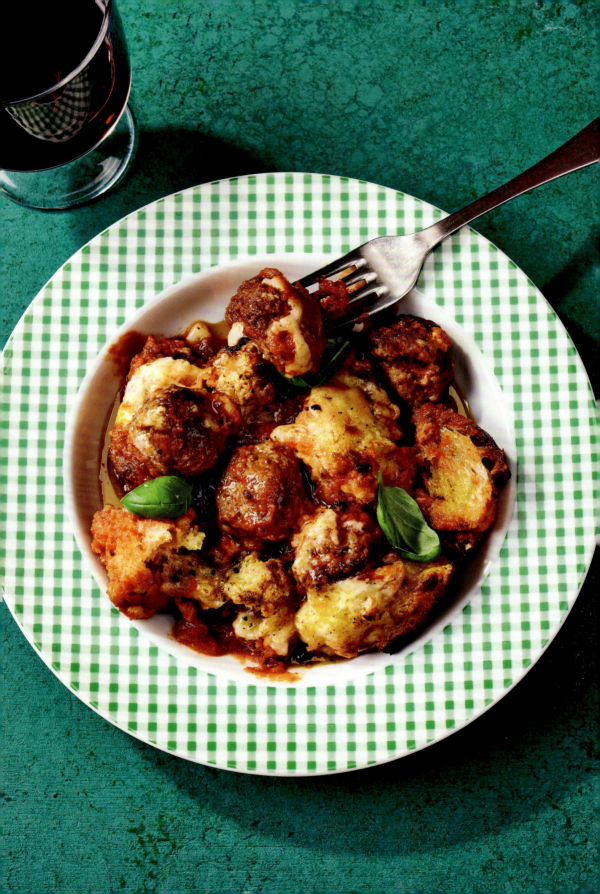

LAZY CHICKEN STROGANOFF

234 CALORIES

SERVES 4

5 MINS

Like many of you, I love a beef stroganoff, but one day I only had chicken and so here we are. This recipe does skip the mushrooms, but feel free to add them if you love them – I sometimes chuck some button mushrooms in whole. A perfect weeknight supper.

400g chicken breasts or thighs, thickly sliced

1½ tbsp Dijon mustard

2 onions, diced

300ml chicken stock

2 heaped tbsp tomato purée or paste (buy one with garlic)

2 tbsp half-fat crème fraîche

1 Add everything to the slow cooker, apart from the crème fraîche. Cook on high for 3–4 hours or low for 6–7 hours.

2 Once cooked, if the sauce is looking thin, add 1–2 tablespoons of cornflour mixed with 1 tablespoon of water to thicken the sauce and cook on high for 30 minutes, then stir in the crème fraîche.

3 Serve.

SERVING NOTE:
Serve with some rice and a little bit of finely chopped fresh parsley.

PROTEIN: 31g | **CARBS:** 19g | **FAT:** 3g

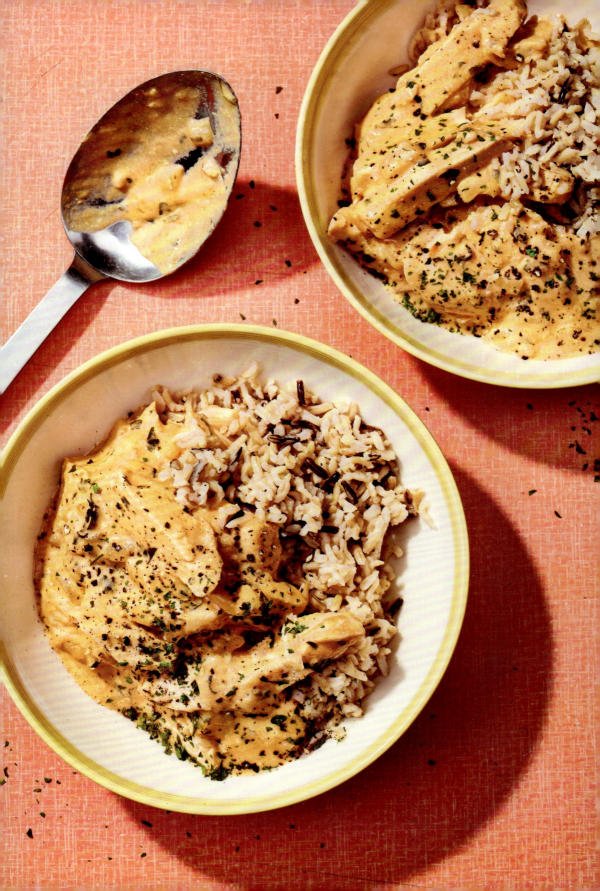

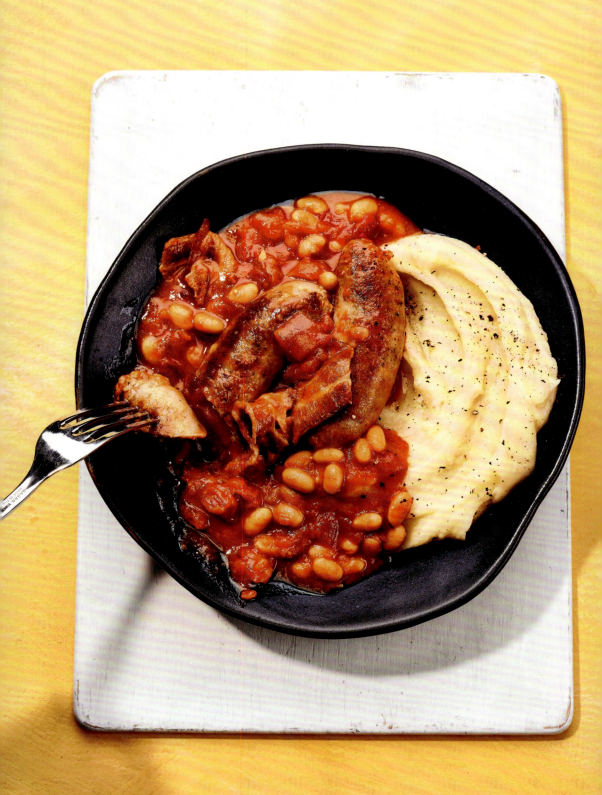

SAUSAGE, BACON & BEAN COWBOY SUPPER

562 CALORIES

SERVES 4

10 MINS

This is the furthest thing from fancy, and it instantly transports me back to my childhood. Having this with a buttery creamy mash on the side, or maybe some greens and buttered bread, is the ultimate childhood nostalgia throwback. This is a simplified version, so feel free to add some herbs, or some spice if you like heat.

8 reduced-fat regular sausages or 32 cocktail sausages

200g smoked streaky bacon rashers, roughly chopped

2 x 400g tins of chopped tomatoes

3 tbsp red pesto

2 tbsp Dijon mustard

2 x 400g tins of baked beans

1 Briefly seal the sausages in a hot frying pan for a few minutes until golden, then remove to a plate and lightly crisp the bacon in the same pan.

2 Add the sausages and bacon to the slow cooker with all the other ingredients, apart from the baked beans, then add some salt and pepper and 150ml of boiling water. Cook on high for 3–4 hours or low for 6–7 hours.

3 For the last 30 minutes, stir in the baked beans, close the lid and heat through.

SERVING NOTE:

This is gorgeous with either chips or mashed potatoes. Kids will love this!

PROTEIN: 36g | **CARBS:** 45g | **FAT:** 23g

STICKY GINGER, PINEAPPLE & THAI BASIL BEEF

316 CALORIES

SERVES 4

10 MINS

This is inspired by some of the travels I have been lucky enough to go on. It was from a street vendor, and it sounded sticky and sweet, so was instantly a yes. This is gorgeous with steamed rice and some greens on the side.

500g lean beef mince

400g tin of pineapple, cut into chunks (reserve and use the liquid from the tin)

2 tbsp garlic and ginger paste

4 tbsp dark soy sauce

handful of fresh Thai basil leaves (regular basil is also fine), plus extra to garnish

1 red chilli, finely chopped, plus extra to garnish

1 Season the mince with salt and pepper, then pan-fry in a little oil (I love sesame oil for this) until browned all over. Add to the slow cooker with all the other ingredients (including the pineapple juice) and cook for 2–3 hours on high or 4–5 hours on low.

2 Serve garnished with extra Thai basil leaves and chopped red chilli.

SERVING NOTE:
Great with rice, some spring onions and lime wedges for squeezing over.

PROTEIN: 28g | **CARBS:** 16g | **FAT:** 16g

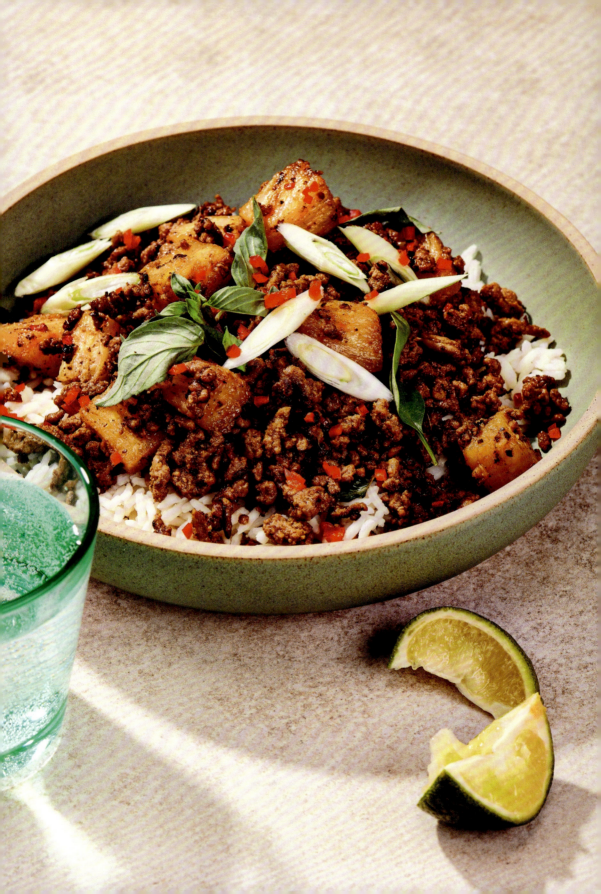

SIMPLE
SWEETS

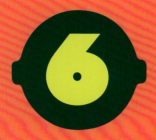

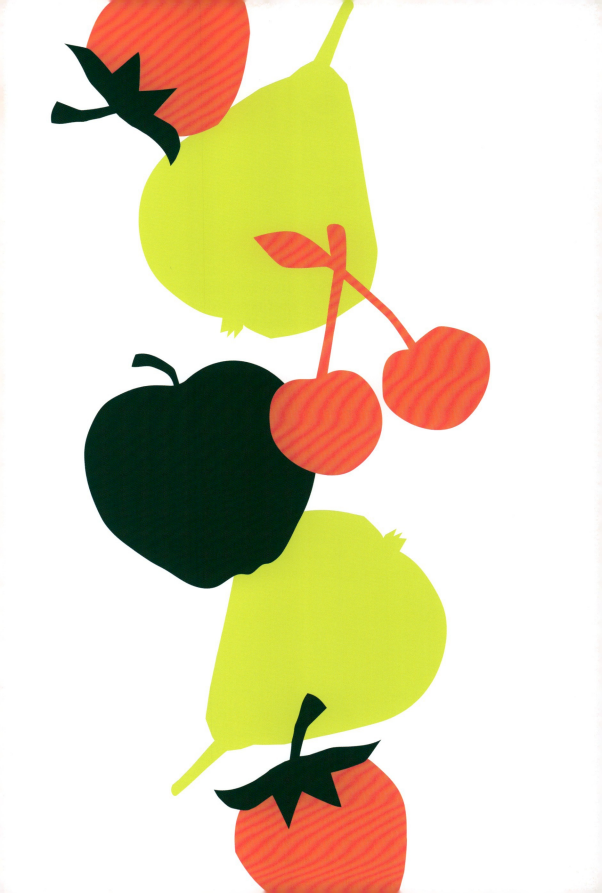

POACHED PEARS

320 CALORIES

SERVES 6

10 MINS

I find it hard to resist a poached pear on a dessert menu, as it just melts in your mouth. This is perfect if you are hosting, and you can use your slow cooker as a backup for dessert. It'll really impress your guests. For an extra treat, serve with cream.

6 pears, peeled and stems left on

2 cinnamon sticks

1 tsp vanilla extract

5 tbsp honey

700ml red wine

150g milk chocolate

1 Add the pears (stems-up) to the slow cooker with all the other ingredients, except the chocolate, and cook on high for 2–3 hours or low for 4–5 hours.

2 For the last 20 minutes or so, grate about 70g of the milk chocolate into the slow cooker so the pears draw in some of that sweetness.

3 Remove the cinnamon sticks. Add the poached pears to bowls or plates and serve with some chocolate shards (see Tips) plus fresh mint leaves, if you like.

TIPS: *Coarsely grate the remaining milk chocolate to make fine shards for serving.*

The sauce left in the slow cooker is reminiscent of mulled wine, so grab yourself a glass!

PROTEIN: 2g | **CARBS:** 36g | **FAT:** 8g

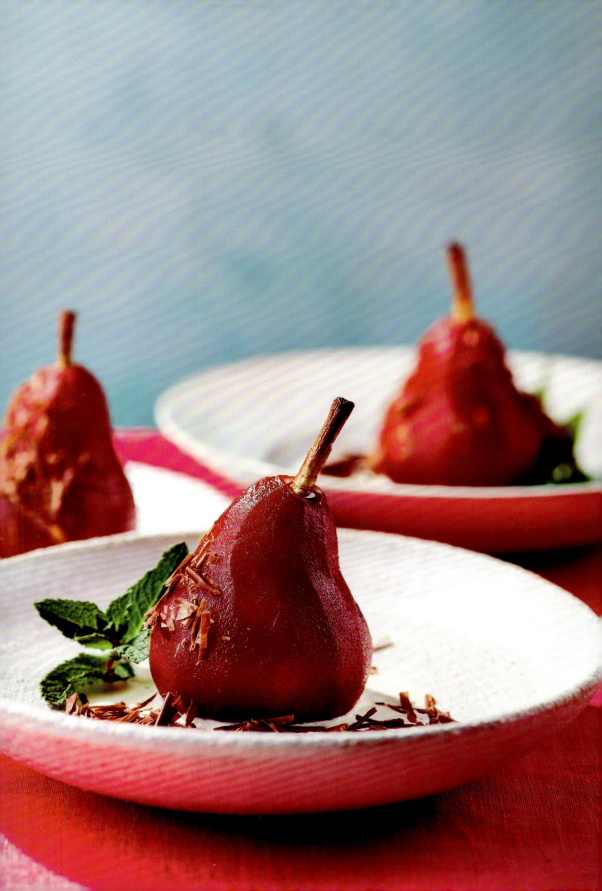

CHOCOLATE FONDANT PUDDING

610 CALORIES

SERVES 6

15 MINS

100g half-fat butter, softened

300g soft light brown sugar

4 eggs, beaten

250g self-raising flour

20g cocoa powder

150g dark chocolate, chopped

This is such a fan-favourite pudding and it couldn't be any easier to make. No one will believe you've cooked it in a slow cooker and the sponge is really airy and light. The star of the show here is definitely the gooey sauce.

1 Firstly, either grease or line your slow cooker with some foil and then baking parchment.

2 Beat together the butter and 150g of the light brown sugar in a bowl until fluffy. Gradually beat in the eggs, then sift over the flour and cocoa powder and gently fold in until combined.

3 Melt 100g of the chocolate and drizzle into the batter with 3–4 tablespoons of water (or milk) so that the batter falls off the spoon in big dollops, then transfer to your lined slow cooker. Spread out evenly with the back of a spoon.

4 Melt the remaining 50g of chocolate and mix with the remaining 150g of sugar and 275ml of boiling water in another bowl until smooth. Drizzle the chocolate liquid all over the cake, cover the slow cooker with a clean tea towel and place on the lid, then cook on high for 2½ hours or on low for 5 hours. Serve hot.

PROTEIN: 11g | **CARBS:** 100g | **FAT:** 20g

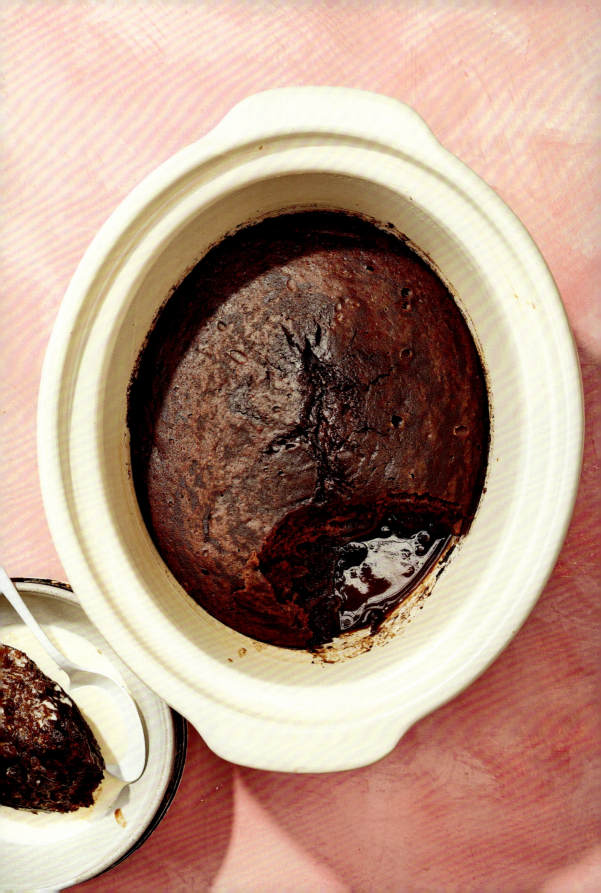

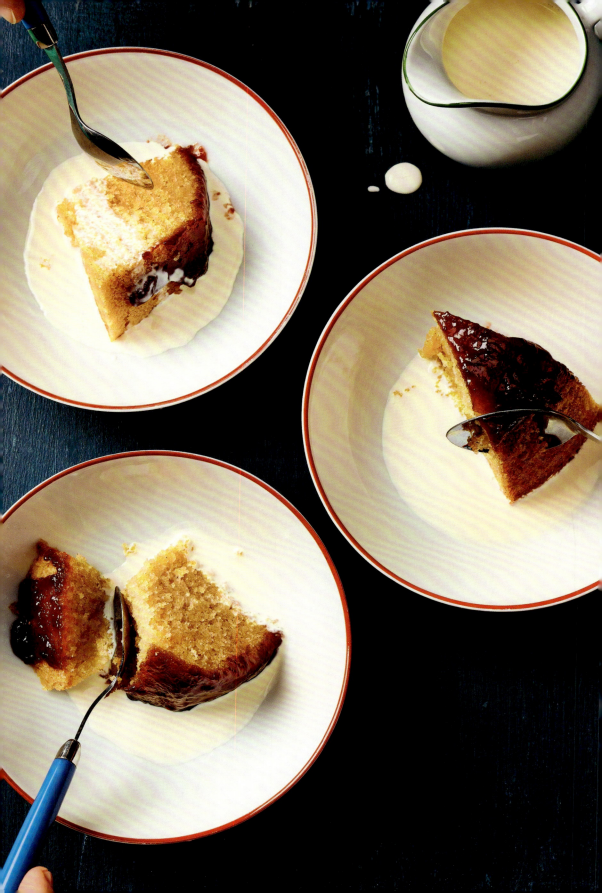

CHERRY JAM STEAMED SPONGE

252 CALORIES

SERVES 6

15 MINS

This is reminiscent of the steamed sponge puddings you had at school, but better. This is true comfort in a bowl and is perfect served with cream or custard. Delicious!

110g half-fat butter, softened, plus extra for greasing

110g caster sugar

110g self-raising flour

2 eggs, beaten

2 tsp vanilla extract

60g cherry jam

1 Grease a large (1 litre) pudding basin or heatproof bowl with butter and line the bottom with greaseproof paper.

2 Beat the butter and sugar together in a bowl until fluffy, then mix in the flour, eggs and vanilla until combined. Add a splash of water or milk to loosen the batter to a dropping consistency.

3 Spread the jam over the base of the prepared basin/bowl and spoon over the batter. Cover the top of the basin tightly with greaseproof paper and foil, then place into the slow cooker on top of a small baking dish or trivet. Pour boiling water around the basin, about 7.5 cm deep. Close the lid and cook on high for 3 hours, or until the sponge is risen and set.

4 To serve, carefully remove the basin from the slow cooker, remove the foil and paper and use a knife to loosen the edges. Place a serving plate over the top and turn the dish over. Remove the basin and use a spoon to scrape out any bits of jam that are still inside. Cut into wedges and serve while warm.

SERVING NOTE:

A good dollop of cream or custard is *chefs kiss* here.

PROTEIN: 4g | **CARBS:** 30g | **FAT:** 8g

DARK CHOCOLATE BROWNIES

182 CALORIES

MAKES 20

10 MINS

Who knew baking was so easy in the slow cooker? These dark chocolate brownies are fudgy and rich – you won't believe how good they are. Enjoy as a warm dessert or leave to cool and keep them as snacks for when you're craving a sweet treat.

200g half-fat butter, diced into cubes

175g dark chocolate, chopped

300g caster sugar

3 eggs, beaten

3 tbsp cocoa powder

80g plain flour

1 Firstly, line your slow cooker with some foil and then baking parchment.

2 Melt the butter and chocolate together in a heatproof bowl in the microwave for 2–3 minutes on high in 30-second bursts (so that the mixture doesn't split), then whisk in the remaining ingredients with a little pinch of salt to make a smooth batter.

3 Spoon the batter into the lined slow cooker, then cover the slow cooker with a clean tea towel and then the lid. Cook on low for 2½–3 hours, then remove the lid and tea towel and cook on low for a 1 further hour, or until the mixture feels set.

4 Remove the brownie from the slow cooker and allow to cool for 5 minutes on a wire rack before cutting into small squares and serving warm or cold.

TIP: *Swirl some salted caramel through the batter before cooking, if you like.*

PROTEIN: 2g | **CARBS:** 24g | **FAT:** 8g

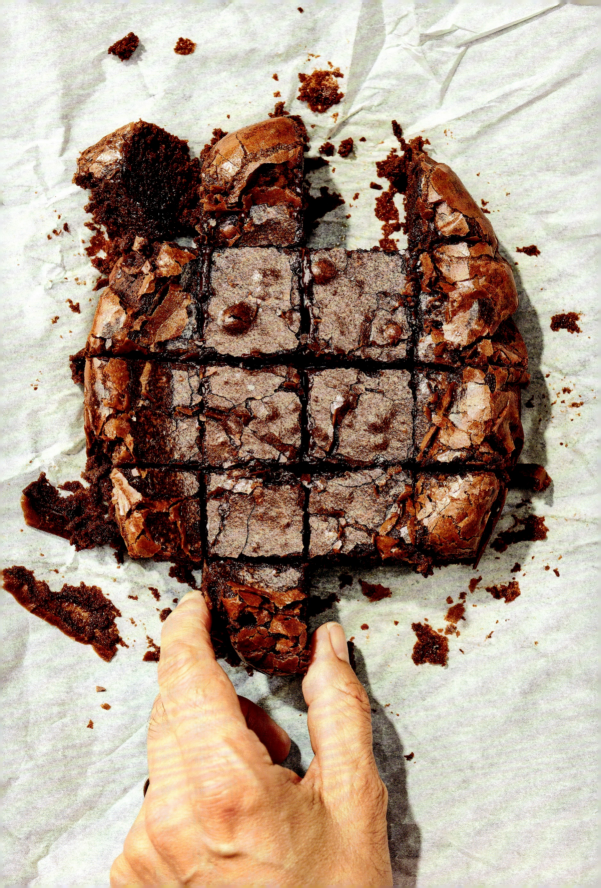

QUEEN OF PUDDINGS

359 CALORIES

SERVES 6

15 MINS

A real showstopper treat of a dessert here and worth the effort, I promise. Not only does it taste incredible, it is super cheap to make. Such simple ingredients, yet something so yummy!

570ml full-fat milk

120g fresh white breadcrumbs

100g caster sugar

50g half-fat butter, melted

3 eggs, separated

200g fruit jam (I like raspberry or blackcurrant)

1 Add the milk, breadcrumbs, 25g of the caster sugar and the melted butter to the slow cooker while it is turned off, and stir well. Allow to sit for 10 minutes so the liquid is fully absorbed.

2 Once absorbed, stir through the egg yolks, then carefully spread the jam over the top. Cook on high for 1 hour or low for 2 hours.

3 When the mixture is nearly ready, whisk the egg whites to stiff peaks and gradually whisk in the remaining 75g of caster sugar until glossy and thick.

4 Spoon the meringue onto the top of the pudding in an even layer and cook on high for another 30 minutes or low for another 1 hour.

5 Just before serving, place the slow cooker pot (make sure it's ovenproof) under a medium grill for a minute or so until the meringue is lightly browned.

SERVING NOTE:
Serving this hot with cream is stunning.

PROTEIN: 10g | **CARBS:** 56g | **FAT:** 10g

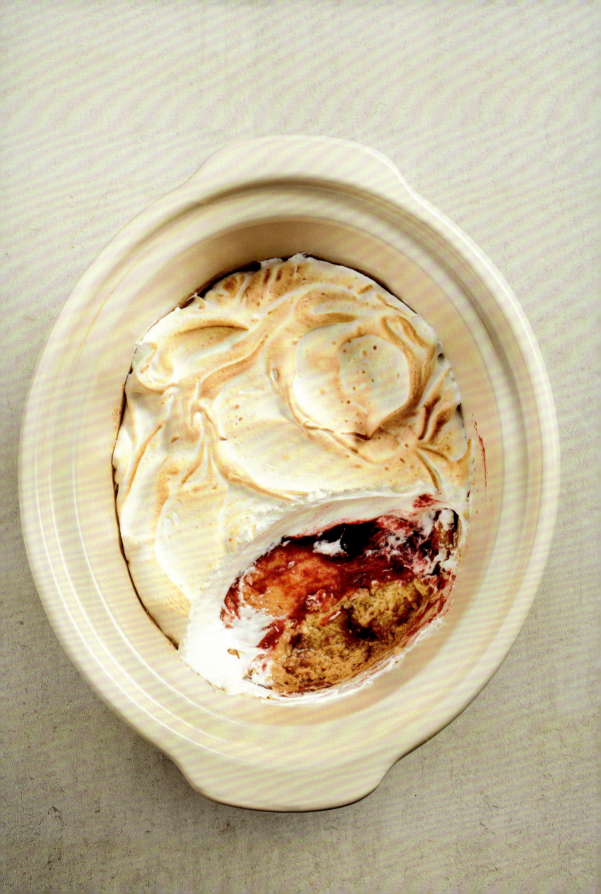

INDEX

Note: page numbers in **bold** refer to illustrations.

B

bacon 11
beef & bacon hotpot 75, **75**
    chicken & bacon pie 56, **57**
    chunky bacon, leek & potato soup 102, **103**
    creamy chicken pasta with mushrooms & bacon **62**, 63
    curried chorizo, bacon & lentil soup 112, **113**
    garlic butter chicken with bacon & sweetcorn 80, **81**
    sausage, bacon & bean cowboy supper **170**, 171
    tartiflette 58, **59**
    tomato, bacon & basil chicken pasta **154**, 155
BBQ honey shredded chicken burgers 126, **127**
bean(s)
    braised bean stew 64, **65**
    chicken & bean white chilli **122**, 123
    chorizo & butter bean soup **92**, 93
    pulled pork & pinto bean chilli with rice 118, **119**
    sausage, bacon & bean cowboy supper **170**, 171
beef
    beef & bacon hotpot 75, **75**
    beef brisket coconut rendang curry 20, **21**
    beef brisket madras 52, **53**
    braised daube of beef in a port gravy 144, **145**
    cheesy beef taco-style rice **130**, 131
    cheesy jalapeño mince 72, **73**
    creamy beef & mushroom orzotto 140, **141**
    easy beef & mushrooms in oyster sauce 26, **27**
    gochujang & BBQ pulled beef 32, **33**
    Irish savoury mince & carrots 136, **137**
    meatball sub bake with crispy croutons 166, **167**
    Philly cheesesteak rolls **22**, 23
    simple steak Diane 69, **69**
    soy & ginger braised short ribs 120, **121**
    sticky chilli mince & noodles 44, **45**
    sticky ginger, pineapple & Thai basil beef 172, **173**
biryani, chicken biryani 16, **17**
breadcrumbs 150, 184
broccoli 110
    broccoli, leek & Stilton soup 96, **97**
brownies, dark chocolate brownies 182, **183**
burgers, honey BBQ shredded chicken burgers 126, **127**

butternut squash, creamy butternut squash & lemon linguine 160, **161**

C

calories 6, 12
carrot 86, 90, 110
    Irish savoury mince & carrots 136, **137**
celery 90, 110
Cheddar cheese 11
    cheesy beef taco-style rice 131
    cheesy jalapeño mince 72, **73**
    meatball sub bake with crispy croutons 166
    Philly cheesesteak rolls 23
cheese
    broccoli, leek & Stilton soup 96, **97**
    chicken & bean white chilli 123
    tartiflette 58
    see also Cheddar cheese; feta; halloumi
cherry jam steamed sponge **180**, 181
chicken 11
    chicken & bacon pie 56, **57**
    chicken & bean white chilli **122**, 123
    chicken & sweetcorn soup **108**, 109
    chicken biryani 16, **17**
    chicken chasni curry 42, **43**
    creamy chicken & potato soup 98, **99**
    creamy chicken meatballs with gnocchi 150, **151**
    creamy chicken pasta with mushrooms & bacon **62**, 63
    creamy white wine chicken **78**, 79
    easy ramen 40, **41**
    garlic butter chicken with bacon & sweetcorn 80, **81**
    honey & sriracha chicken 24, **25**
    honey BBQ shredded chicken burgers 126, **127**
    lazy chicken stroganoff 168, **169**
    lemon, black pepper & butter chicken **162**, 163
    marry me chicken made easy 148, **149**
    pesto & sundried tomato chicken **70**, 71
    sticky hoisin & orange chicken legs **38**, 39
    takeaway-inspired garlic pepper chicken 34, **35**
    tomato, bacon & basil chicken pasta **154**, 155
    whole vindaloo chicken & potatoes 132, **133**
chickpea

chickpea, potato & chorizo stew 156, **157**
lamb & chickpea stew with couscous 60, **61**
chilli (dish)
chicken & bean white chilli **122**, 123
pulled pork & pinto bean chilli with rice 118, **119**
chocolate
chocolate fondant pudding 178, **179**
dark chocolate brownies 182, **183**
poached pears 176, **177**
chorizo 10
chickpea, potato & chorizo stew 156, **157**
chorizo & butter bean soup **92**, 93
curried chorizo, bacon & lentil soup 112, **113**
harissa & chorizo shakshuka 104, **105**
coconut milk (reduced-fat)
beef brisket coconut rendang curry 20, **21**
beef brisket madras 52, **53**
duck legs & pineapple curry 48, **49**
king prawn curry 28
pork shoulder Thai green curry 50, **51**
red Thai curry soup 88, **89**
rogan josh pulled pork curry **30**, 31
whole vindaloo chicken & potatoes 132
cod, lemon paprika cod **138**, 139
couscous, lamb & chickpea stew with couscous 60,
61
cream cheese, chicken & bean white chilli 123
cream (double) 10
crème fraîche 10
croutons, crispy croutons 166, **167**
curry
beef brisket coconut rendang curry 20, **21**
beef brisket madras 52, **53**
black lentil dahl **100**, 101
chicken biryani 16, **17**
chicken chasni curry 42, **43**
curried chorizo, bacon & lentil soup 112, **113**
curried lentils & leeks 106, **107**
duck legs & pineapple curry 48, **49**
king prawn curry 28, **29**
lamb keema 46, **47**
pork shoulder Thai green curry 50, **51**
red Thai curry soup 88, **89**
rogan josh pulled pork curry **30**, 31

sausage currywurst 36, **37**
whole vindaloo chicken & potatoes 132, **133**

D
dahl, black lentil dahl **100**, 101
defrosting food 12
duck
duck legs & pineapple curry 48, **49**
duck pilaf 152, **153**

E
egg, harissa & chorizo shakshuka 104, **105**

F
feta, tomato & red pepper pasta 164, **165**
fish, lemon paprika cod **138**, 139
freezing food 12

G
garlic
garlic butter chicken with bacon & sweetcorn 80, **81**
takeaway-inspired garlic pepper chicken 34, **35**
ginger
soy & ginger braised short ribs 120, **121**
sticky ginger, pineapple & Thai basil beef 172, **173**
gnocchi, creamy chicken meatballs with gnocchi 150,
151
gochujang
gochujang & BBQ pulled beef 32, **33**
gochujang honey ribs 158, **159**
gravy, port gravy 144, **145**

H
halloumi, spiced sweet potato & halloumi soup 86, **87**
ham hock & split pea soup 90, **91**
harissa
harissa & chorizo shakshuka 104, **105**
harissa lamb sliders 116, **117**
hoisin sauce, sticky hoisin & orange chicken legs **38**,
39
honey
gochujang honey ribs 158, **159**

Index

honey & sriracha chicken 24, **25**
honey BBQ shredded chicken burgers 126, **127**
hotpot, beef & bacon hotpot 75, **75**

J

jalapeño(s), cheesy jalapeño mince 72, **73**

K

keema, lamb keema 46, **47**

L

lamb
　harissa lamb sliders 116, **117**
　lamb & chickpea stew with couscous 60, **61**
　lamb with balsamic vinegar 124, **125**
　lamb keema 46, 4**7**
　Sunday roast lamb 134, **135**
leek 98, 110
　broccoli, leek & Stilton soup 96, **97**
　chunky bacon, leek & potato soup 102, **103**
　curried lentils & leeks 106, **107**
lemon
　creamy butternut squash & lemon linguine 160, **161**
　lemon, black pepper & butter chicken **162**, 163
　lemon paprika cod **138**, 139
lentil(s)
　black lentil dahl **100**, 101
　curried chorizo, bacon & lentil soup 112, **113**
　curried lentils & leeks 106, **107**
　sweet potato & lentil shepherd's pie 142, **143**
linguine, creamy butternut squash & lemon linguine
　160, **161**

M

madras, beef brisket madras 52, **53**
mangetout 50, 88
meatballs
　creamy chicken meatballs with gnocchi 150, **151**
　meatball sub bake with crispy croutons 166, **167**
　winter sausage meatballs & cream 66, **67**
mince, cheesy jalapeño mince 72, **73**
mushroom 82
　creamy beef & mushroom orzotto 140, **141**

creamy chicken pasta with mushrooms & bacon
　62, 63
　easy beef & mushrooms in oyster sauce 26, **27**
rich pork sausage & porcini ragù 82, **83**

N

noodles 94
　easy ramen 40, **41**
　sticky chilli mince & noodles 44, **45**

O

orzotto, creamy beef & mushroom orzotto 140, **141**
oyster sauce with easy beef & mushroms 26, **27**

P

pantry essentials 8
pasta
　creamy beef & mushroom orzotto 140, **141**
　creamy butternut squash & lemon linguine 160, **161**
　creamy chicken pasta with mushrooms & bacon
　　62, 63
　creamy pork sausage pasta 76, **77**
　feta, tomato & red pepper pasta 164, **165**
　tomato, bacon & basil chicken pasta **154**, 155
pear, poached pears 176, **177**
pepper 88, 118, 131
　feta, tomato & red pepper pasta 164, **165**
pesto 76, 171
　pesto & sundried tomato chicken **70**, 71
　pesto & prosciutto pork with potatoes 128, **129**
pies
　chicken & bacon pie 56, **57**
　sweet potato & lentil shepherd's pie 142, **143**
pilaf, duck pilaf 152, **153**
pineapple
　duck legs & pineapple curry 48, **49**
　sticky ginger, pineapple & Thai basil beef 172, **173**
pork
　creamy pork sausage pasta 76, **77**
　gochujang honey ribs 158, 1**59**
　meatball sub bake with crispy croutons 166, **167**
　pesto & prosciutto pork with potatoes 128, **129**
　pork shoulder Thai green curry 50, **51**
　pulled pork & pinto bean chilli with rice 118, **119**
　rich pork sausage & porcini ragù 82, **83**

rogan josh pulled pork curry **30**, 31
sticky chilli mince & noodles 44, **45**
tangy lemongrass pork 18, **19**
port gravy 144, **145**
potato 58, 64, 75, 110
    chickpea, potato & chorizo stew 156, **157**
    chunky bacon, leek & potato soup 102, **103**
    creamy chicken & potato soup 98, **99**
    pesto & prosciutto pork with potatoes 128, **129**
    whole vindaloo chicken & potatoes 132, **133**
prawn
    ginger, pak choi & prawn soup 94, **95**
    king prawn curry 28, **29**
prosciutto & pesto pork with potatoes 128, **129**
puddings
    chocolate fondant pudding 178, **179**
    queen of puddings 184, 1**85**

Q
queen of puddings 184, **185**

R
ragù, rich pork sausage & porcini ragù 82, **83**
rendang, beef brisket coconut rendang curry 20, **21**
ribs
    gochujang honey ribs 158, **159**
    soy & ginger braised short ribs 120, **121**
rice
    cheesy beef taco-style rice **130**, 131
    chicken biryani 16, **17**
    duck pilaf 152, **153**
    pulled pork & pinto bean chilli with rice 118, **119**
rogan josh pulled pork curry **30**, 31

S
sausage
    bacon & bean cowboy supper **170**, 171
    sausage currywurst 36, **37**
    winter sausage meatballs & cream 66, **67**
shakshuka, harissa & chorizo shakshuka 104, **105**
shepherd's pie, sweet potato & lentil shepherd's pie
    142, **143**
sliders, harissa lamb sliders 116, **117**
slow cooker kit 9

soup
    broccoli, leek & Stilton soup 96, **97**
    chicken & sweetcorn soup **108**, 109
    chorizo & butter bean soup **92**, 93
    chunky bacon, leek & potato soup 102, **103**
    creamy chicken & potato soup 98, **99**
    curried chorizo, bacon & lentil soup 112, **113**
    ginger, pak choi & prawn soup 94, **95**
    ham hock & split pea soup 90, **91**
    loaded vegetable soup 110, **111**
    red Thai curry soup 88, **89**
    spiced sweet potato & halloumi soup 86, **87**
soy & ginger braised short ribs 120, **121**
spinach 66, 93, 156
split pea & ham hock soup 90, **91**
sponge, cherry jam steamed sponge **180**, 181
sriracha & honey chicken 24, **25**
stew
    braised bean stew 64, **65**
    chickpea, potato & chorizo stew 156, **157**
    lamb & chickpea stew with couscous 60, **61**
sticky chilli mince & noodles 44, **45**
sticky ginger, pineapple & Thai basil beef 172, **173**
sticky hoisin & orange chicken legs **38**, 39
stroganoff, lazy chicken stroganoff 168, **169**
sweet potato
    spiced sweet potato & halloumi soup 86, **87**
    sweet potato & lentil shepherd's pie 142, **143**
sweetcorn
    chicken & sweetcorn soup **108**, 109
    garlic butter chicken with bacon & sweetcorn 80, **81**

T
taco-style rice, cheesy beef taco-style rice **130**, 131

tartiflette 58, **59**
tomato 46, 52, 64, 104, 131, 142, 148, 171
    feta, tomato & red pepper pasta 164, **165**
    pesto & sundried tomato chicken **70**, 71
    tomato, bacon & basil chicken pasta **154**, 155
    tomato passata 31–2, 36, 42, 82, 101, 112, 118, 150,
      166

V
vindaloo, whole vindaloo chicken & potatoes 132, **133**

THANKS

First of all, thanks to every single person who has ever bought one of my cookbooks and followed my journey as a home cook. If this is your first BOL cookbook, then hello and thank you so much for snapping this up. It genuinely means so much to me, you have no idea.

To my incredible publishing team at Ebury and all of my international publishers across the globe. Thank you for taking an Irish home cook and bringing me into so many homes across the world. I think my books have been translated into over 8 languages now, which is so mind-blowing.

To all of my amazing friends and family who have supported me from Day 1, I love you all dearly and would be lost without your never-ending support.

To the people who helped bring this book to life: Celia Palazzo, Steph Milner, Liv Nightingall, Steph Reynolds, Alice King, Lara McLeod, Francesca Thomson, Nikki Dupin, Dan Jones, Natalie Thomson, Max Robinson, Caitlin MacDonald, Hattie Baker, Sam Duff and Lauren Wall. Thank you!!!

To Natalie and the team at *This Morning*, for welcoming me in and making a home cook feel so at ease on national television.

To my management team: Lois, Lucy, Guy, Cara, Simona and Amanda, for pushing me to work outside my comfort zone and believing in me!

I'm very lucky to have all of these people around me, especially all of you readers at home.

Thank you,

Nathan

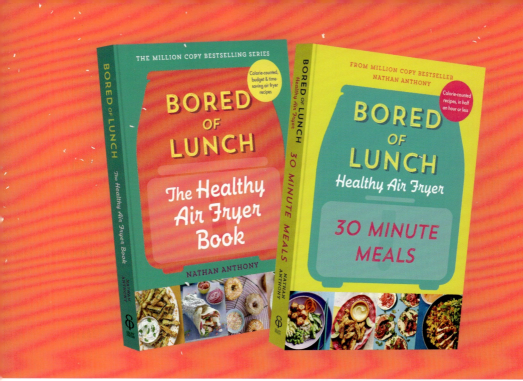

ALSO FROM

BORED OF LUNCH

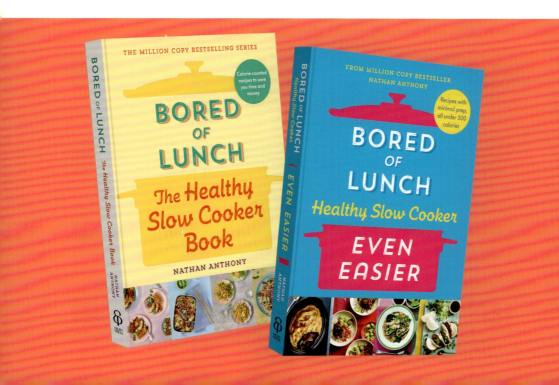

1

Ebury Press, an imprint of Ebury Publishing
One Embassy Gardens, 8 Viaduct Gdns,
Nine Elms, London, SW11 7BW

Ebury Press is part of the Penguin Random House group of companies whose addresses can be found
at global.penguinrandomhouse.com

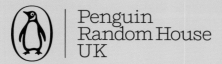

Penguin
Random House
UK

First published by Ebury Press in 2024
www.penguin.co.uk
A CIP catalogue record for this book is available from the British Library

Hardback ISBN 978 1 529 91449 8
Ebook ISBN 978 1 529 91450 4

Publishing Director: Steph Milner
Senior Commissioning Editor: Celia Palazzo
Senior Editor: Liv Nightingall
Production Director: Catherine Ngwong
Design: Nikki Dupin for Studio Nic&Lou
Photography: Dan Jones
Food Stylist: Natalie Thomson
Prop Stylist: Max Robinson

Printed and bound in Italy by LEGO SpA
Colour origination by Altaimage

The authorised representative in the EEA is Penguin Random House Ireland, Morrison Chambers, 32
Nassau Street, Dublin D02 YH68.

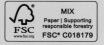

Penguin Random House is committed to a sustainable future for our business,
our readers and our planet. This book is made from Forest Stewardship Council®
certified paper.